# The Swan Kid
## Syndrome Without A Name

I0106585

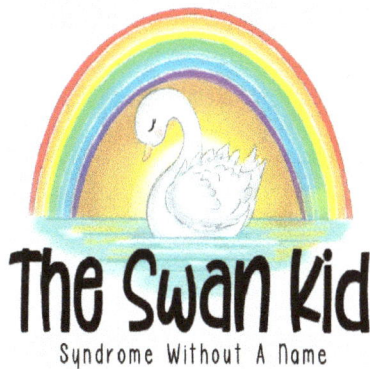

This book is dedicated to all children with or without a disability. Everyone is born with the ability to love, respect and be kind. We are not all the same and that is okay.

~ This book is inspired by my son Antonio Luis, born with an unkown rare genetic syndrome. He is my motivation and reason to keep searching for an answer. ~

The inspiration behind these characters are family to me and I love dearly. Emmanuel my nephew, Jecenia my niece thanks to my sisters Madelyn and Jessica for raising these amazing special children. Thank you to my best friend Tiffany known as Mrs. Rosie in the book, for dedicating your life to Education and helping those with Special Needs.

To my husband Oscar and children Ashley and Ethan. I want to thank you for the love and help you have given Aj and I. Thank you to my mom for whom we are extremely grateful for.

Thank you to all the family, friends that have become family and give endless support. For more dedications please check out our website.

www.theswankids.com

# The day was finally here
## Aj woke up so happy.

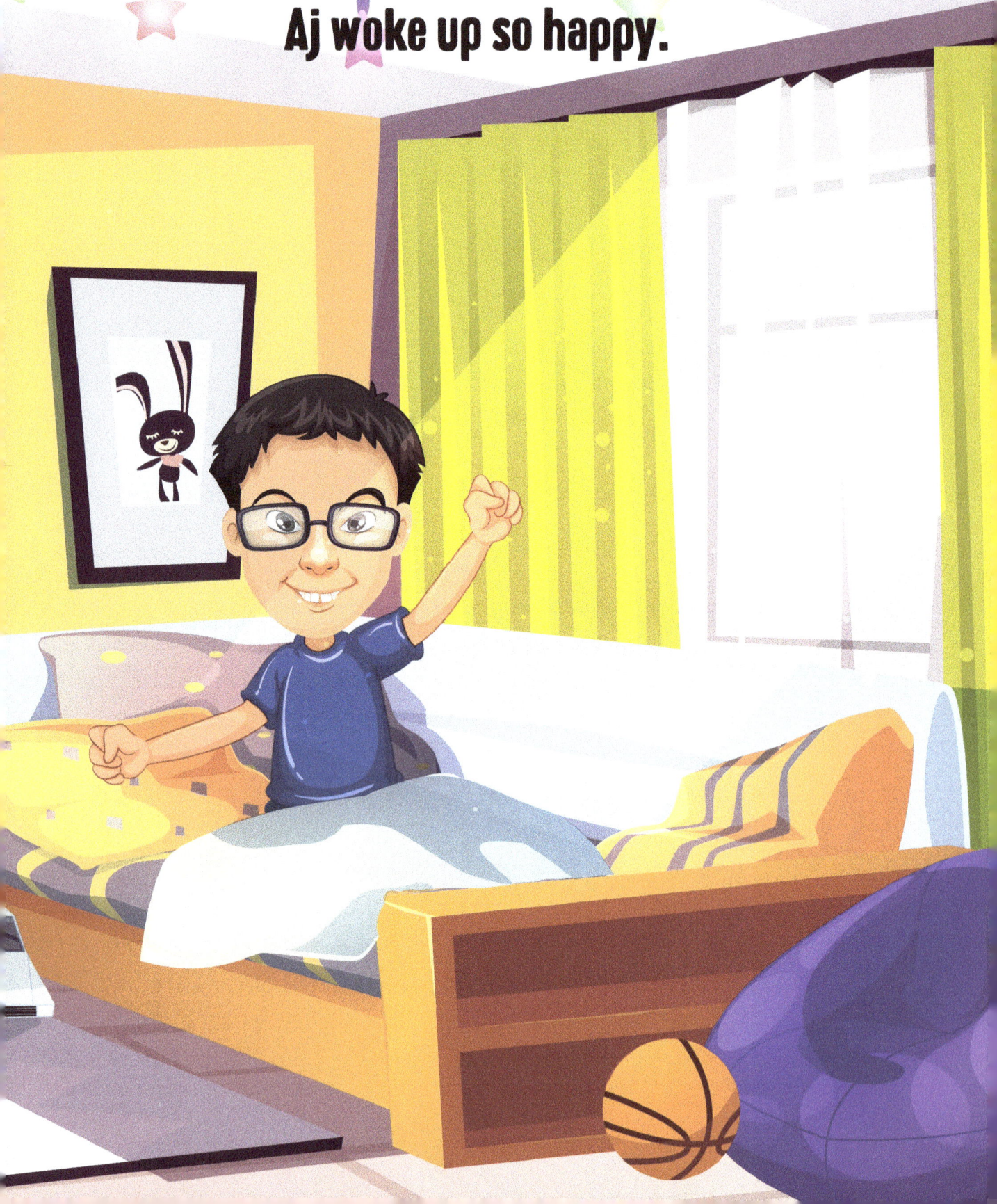

Aj ran down the stairs letting everyone know that today he will be leaving for sleep away camp.

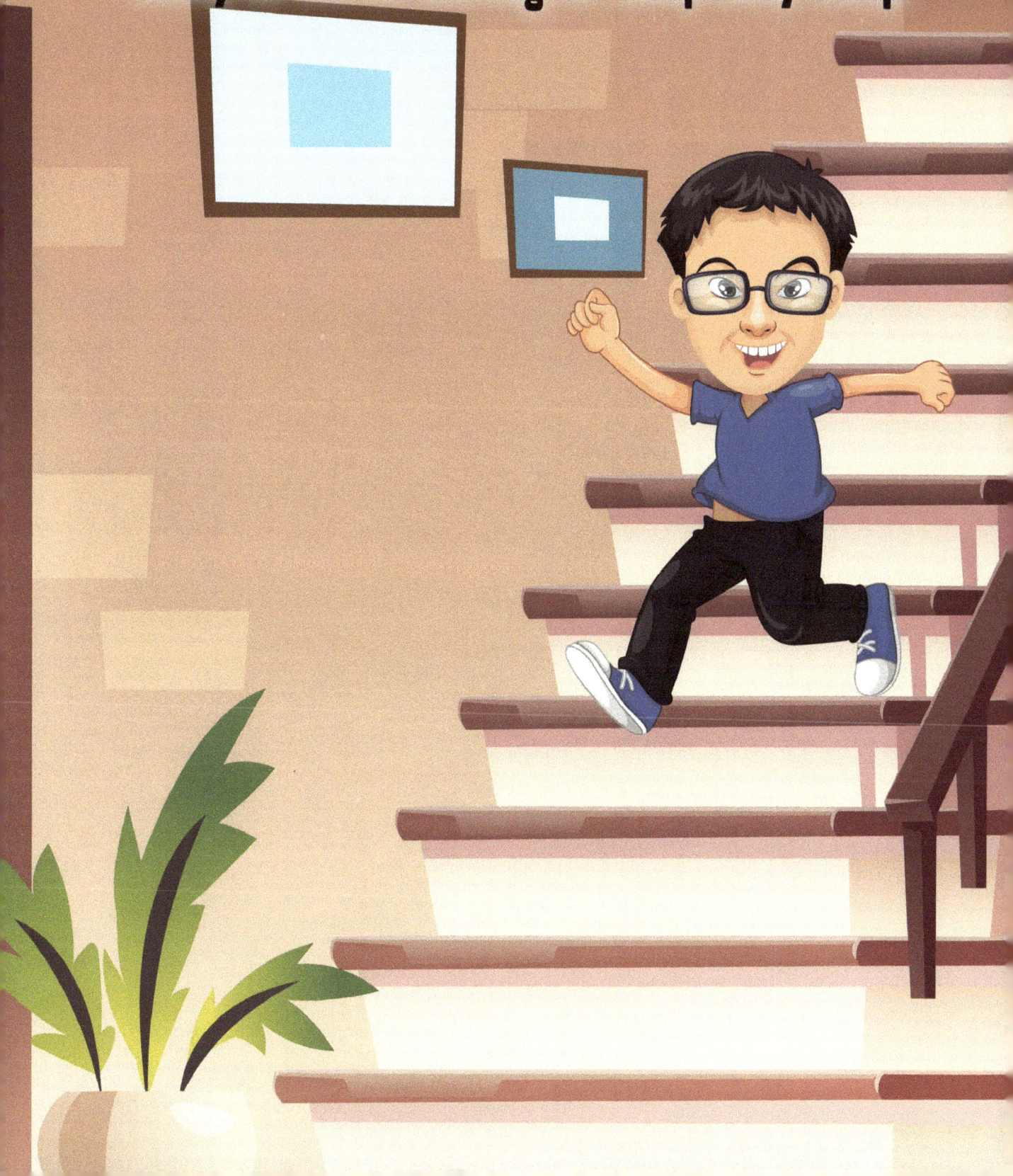

Ethan began to tease Aj about being scared at night. Ethan was just being a big brother but deep down inside we knew he was sad because he was going to miss Aj.

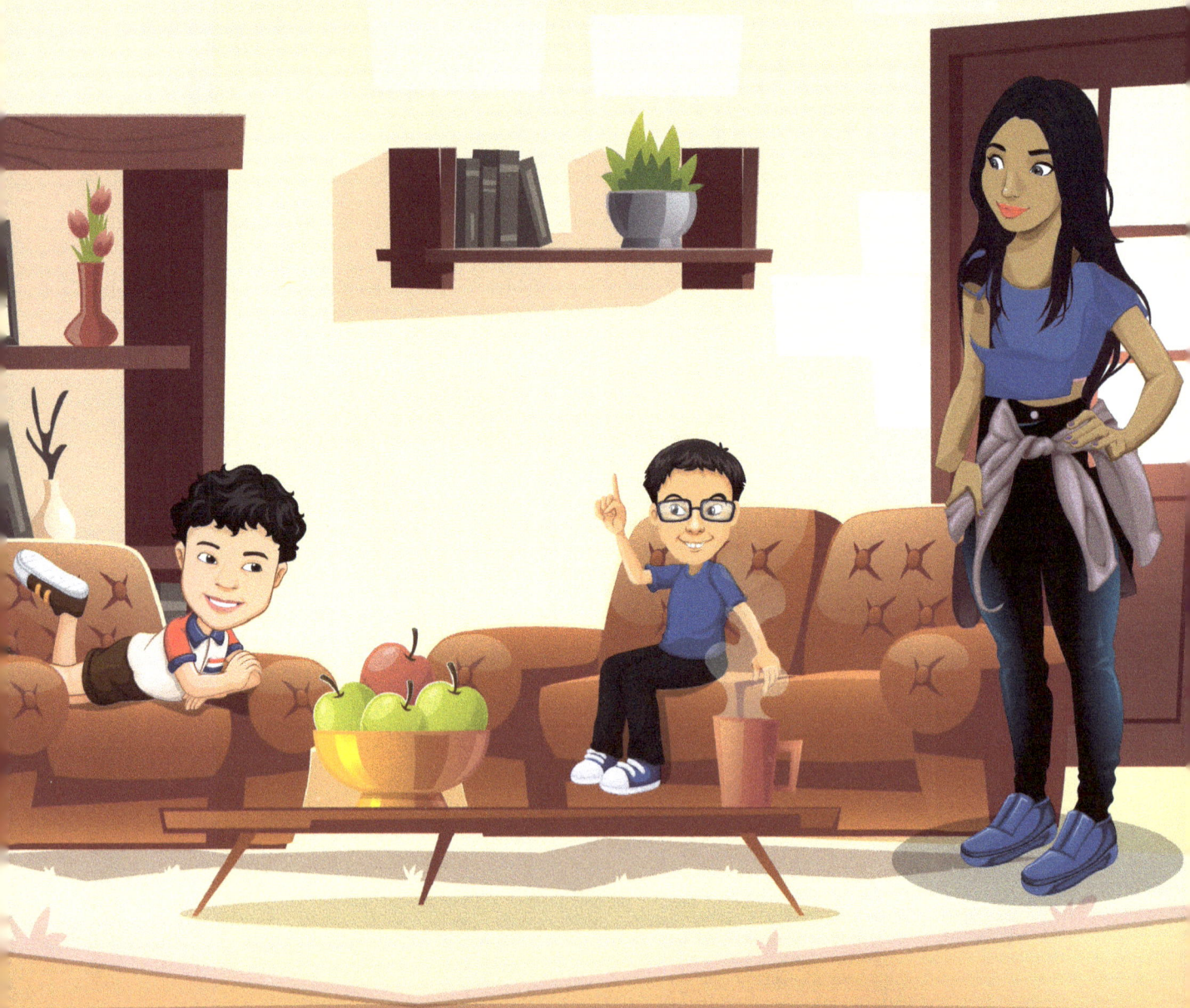

Aj was dressed and ready to go. He met his best friend outside.
Her name is Imani and she lives across the street.

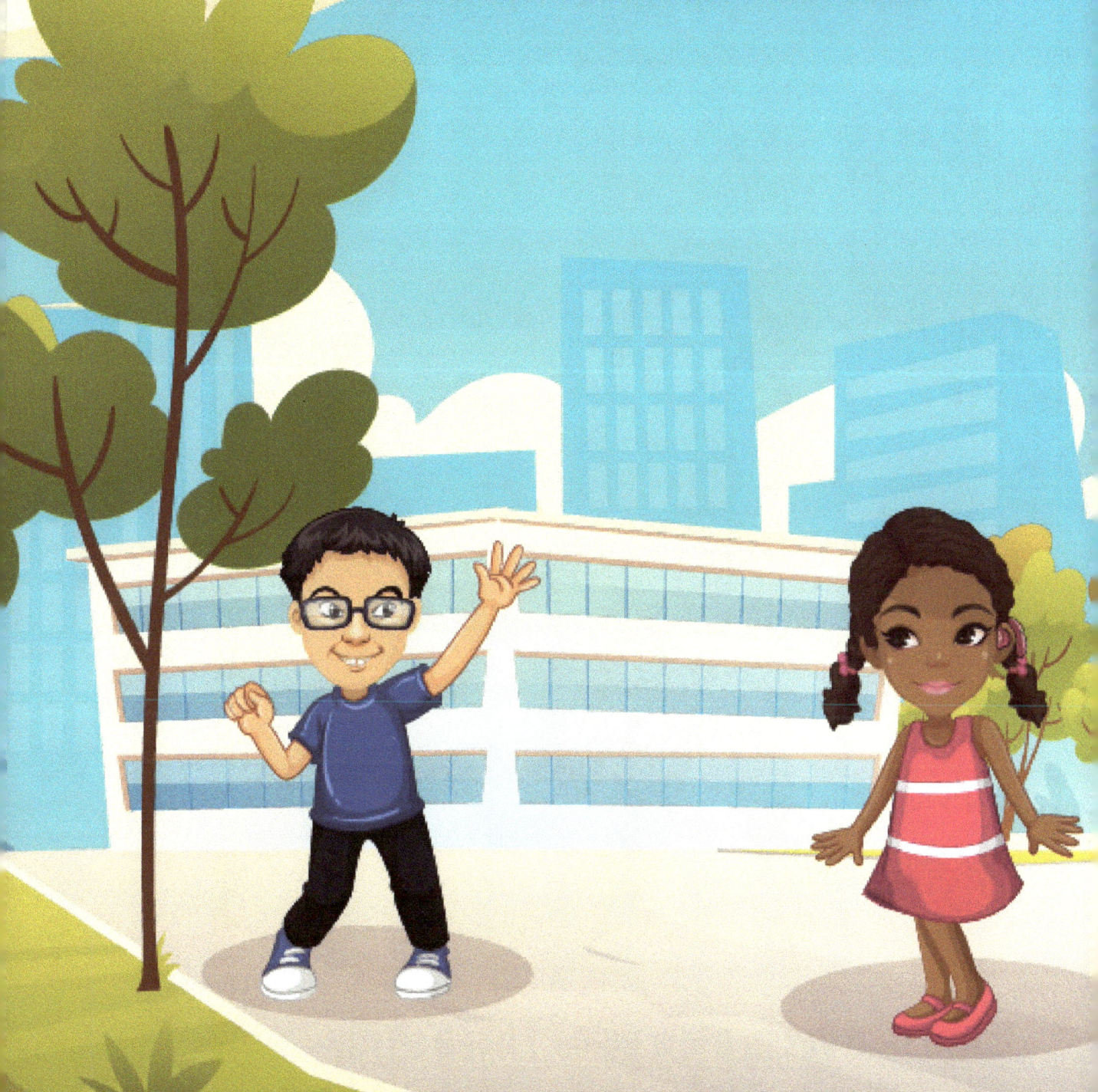

Finally I'm 7 years old and can go to camp, said Aj.
Imani are you ready to go to the camp?

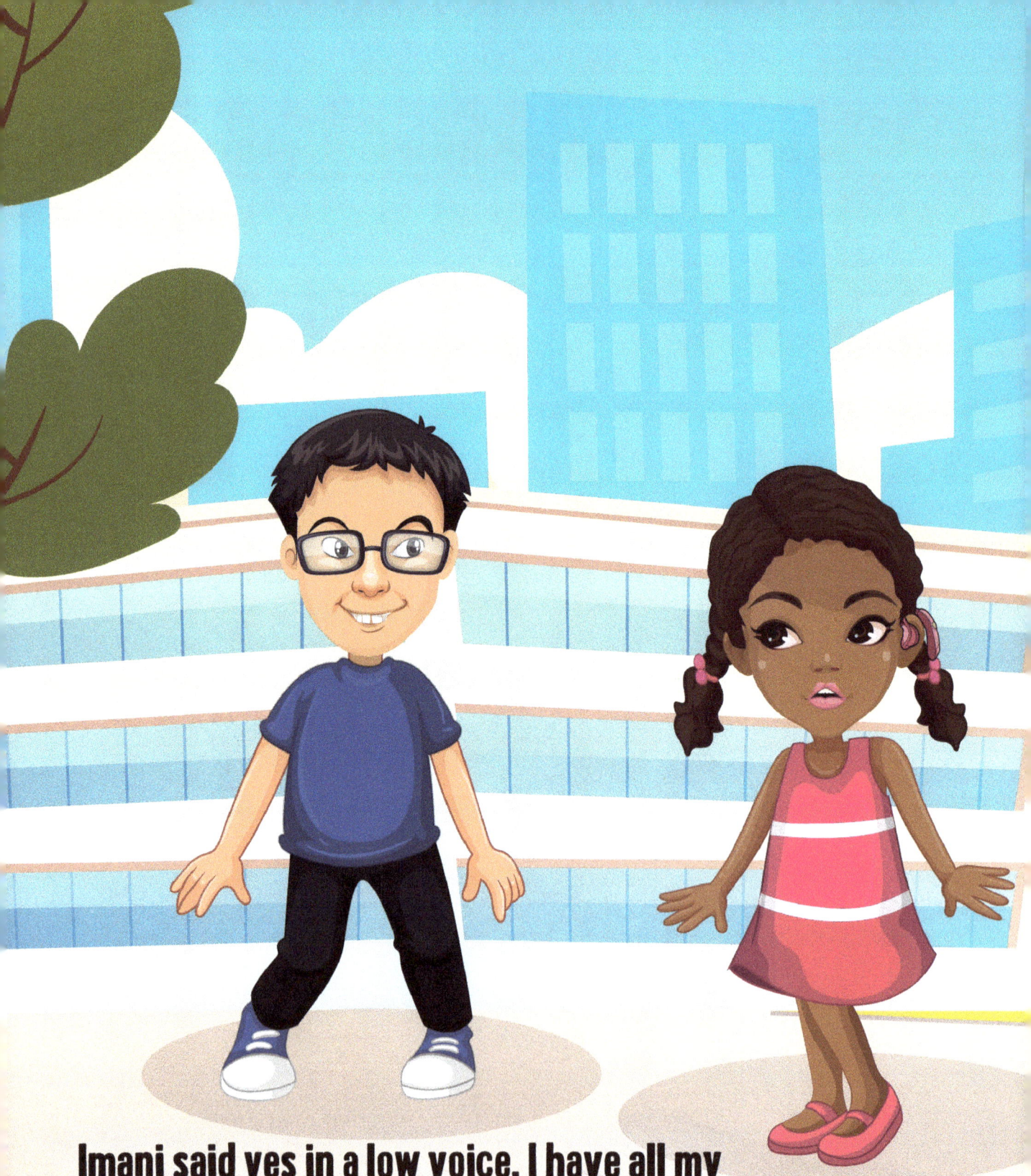

Imani said yes in a low voice. I have all my things but I don't know if I am ready. I hope I can make friends and no one is mean to me.

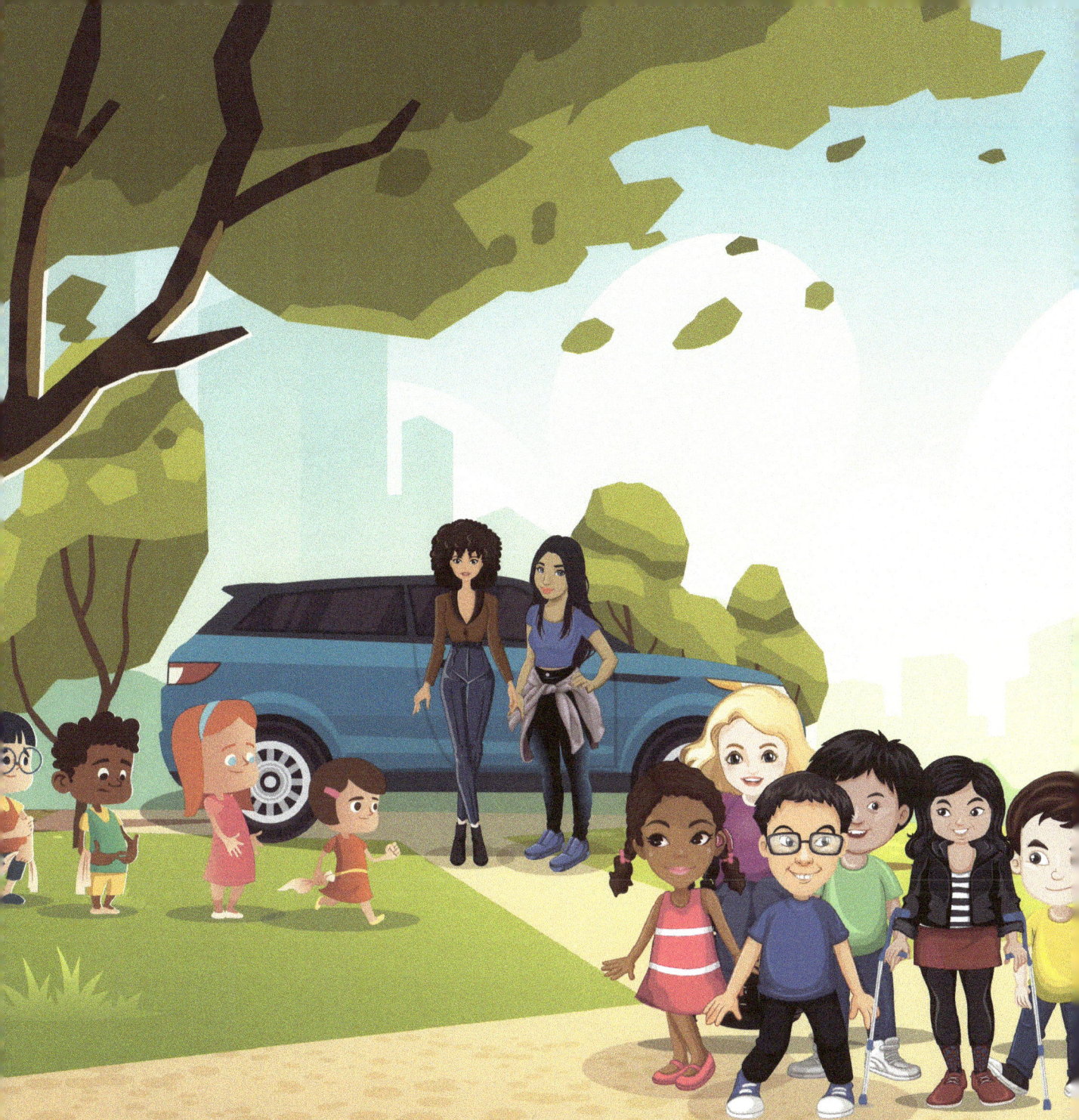

The mothers of Aj and Imani drive them to summer camp.
When they arrive all the kids line up in their groups
by their age.
It took Aj no time to find his group at all.

Mrs. Rosie was the teacher for Aj's group and she wanted everyone to learn about each other. She asked all the kids to name one super power and one weakness that they have.

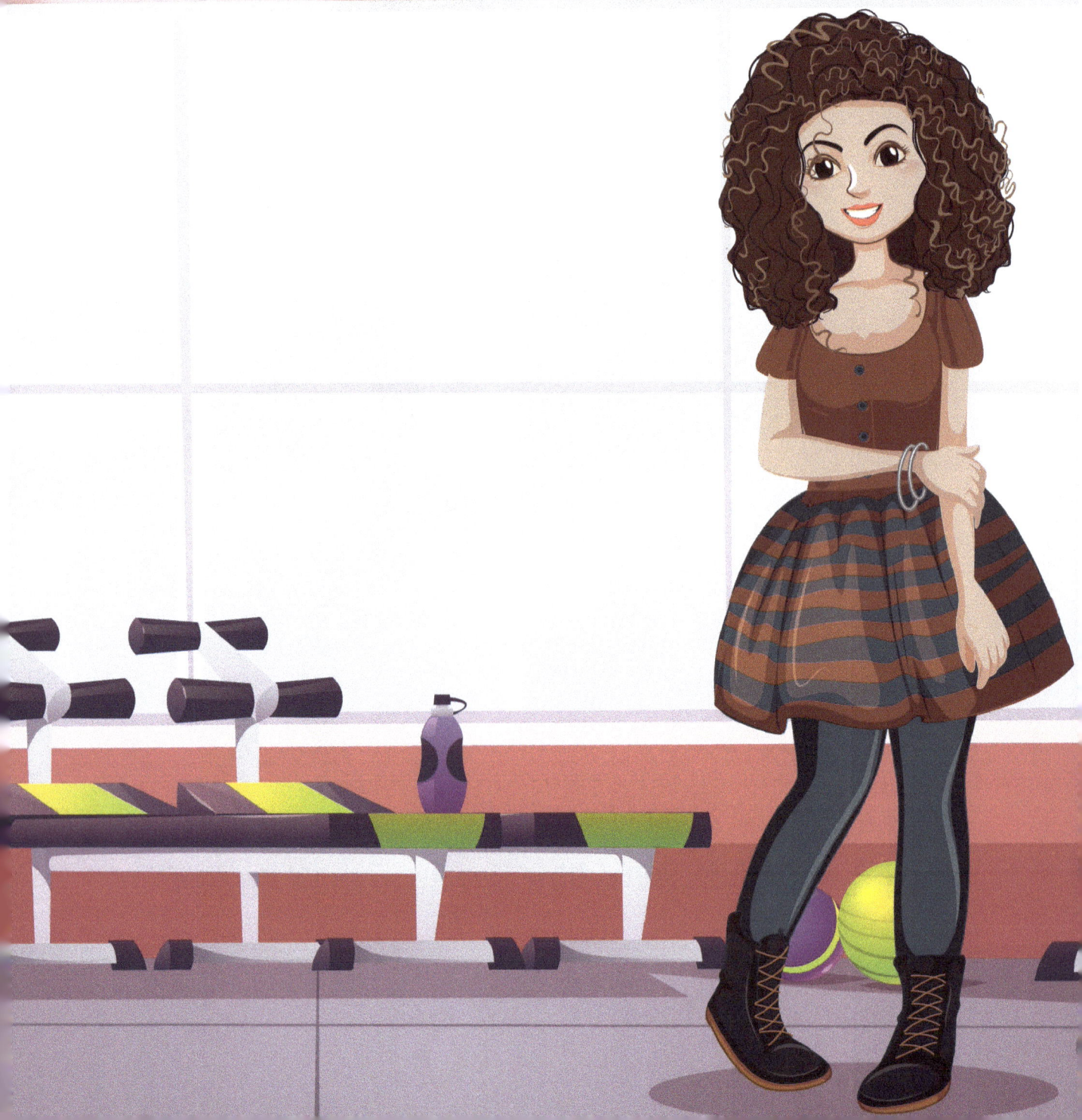

Danny jumped up first and said I have superpowers.
I love music and dancing is my super power.
Weakness Hmm... I don't know how to answer that
but may be it's the way I talk because I have Down Syndrome
I have a hard time using my words and that makes its hard for
people to understand me.

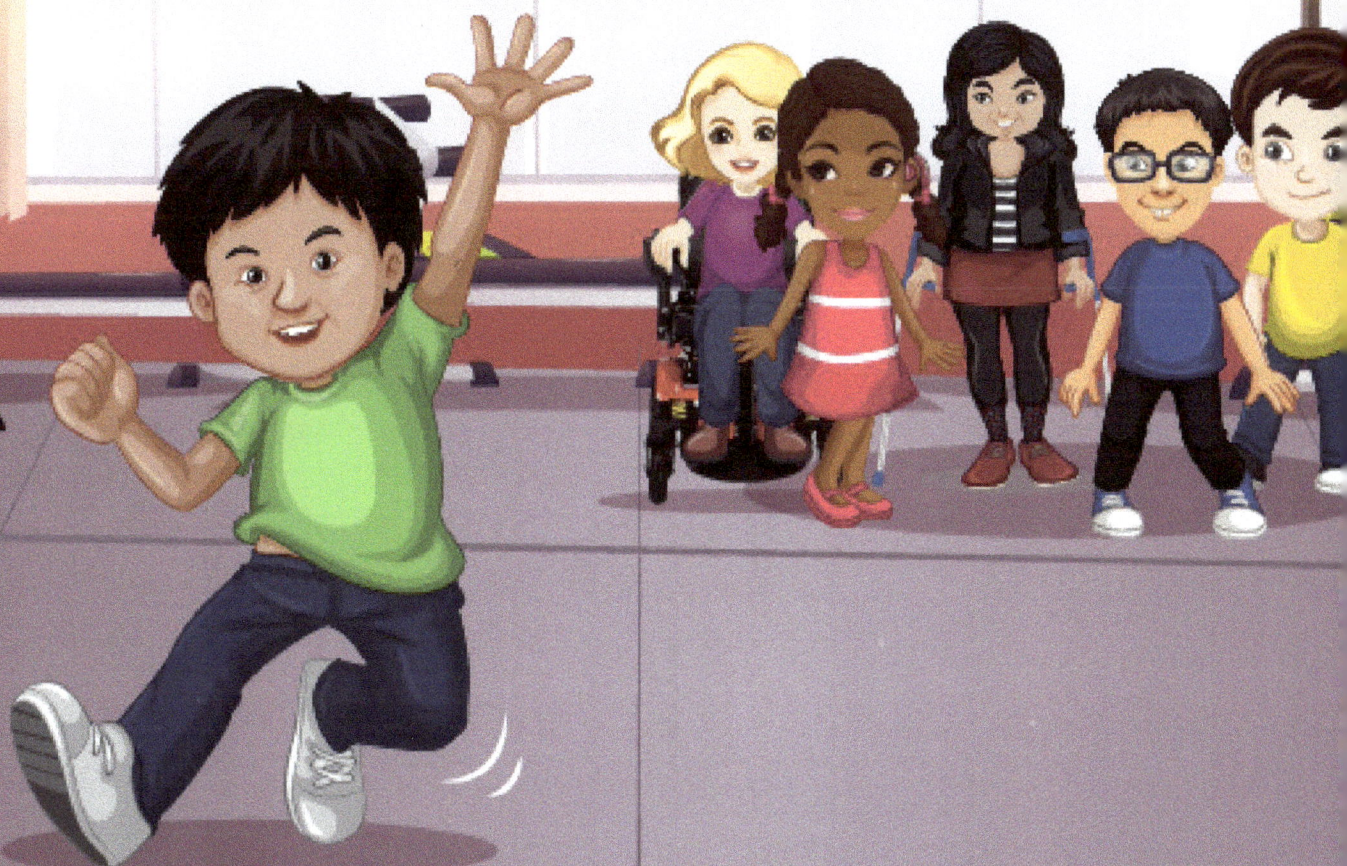

Next was Imani  she said softly that her super power and her weakness both come from her hearing loss.
She showed off her hearing aid and said
"I was born deaf."
My superpower is that I learned how to use all my other senses. My weakness is only being able to hear with a machine.

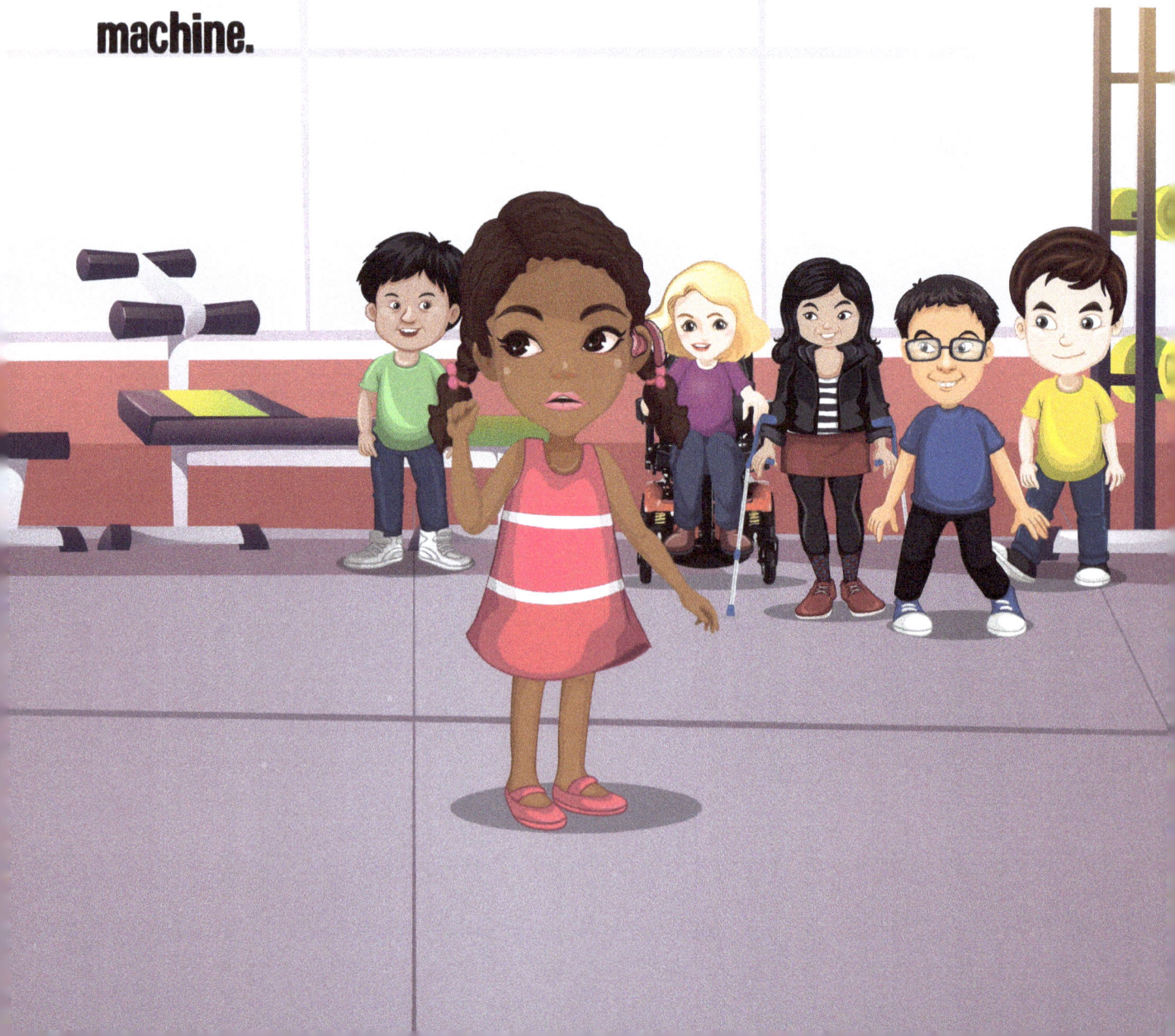

Jesse short for Jecenia was not shy at all. She stood tall and proud then said "my superpower is to walk and talk." I can do a lot of things said Jesse with a big smile. My weakness is that I need more help doing things than other kids, but not so bad for someone with Cerebral Palsy.

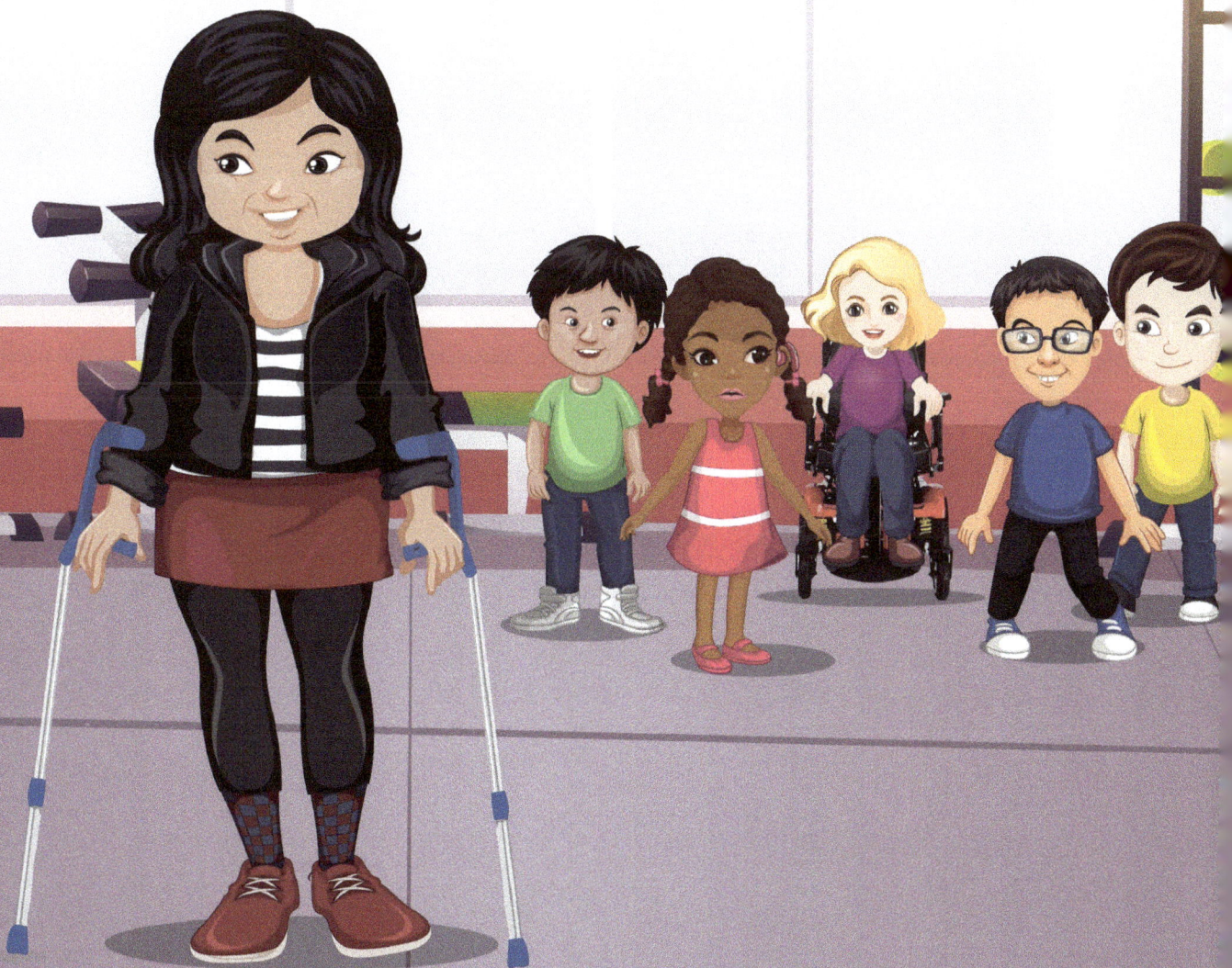

Aj was not sure at this point what to say. He was happy, a little nervous. Aj was shaking and looking around. He realized there were only two kids left so he better get ready.

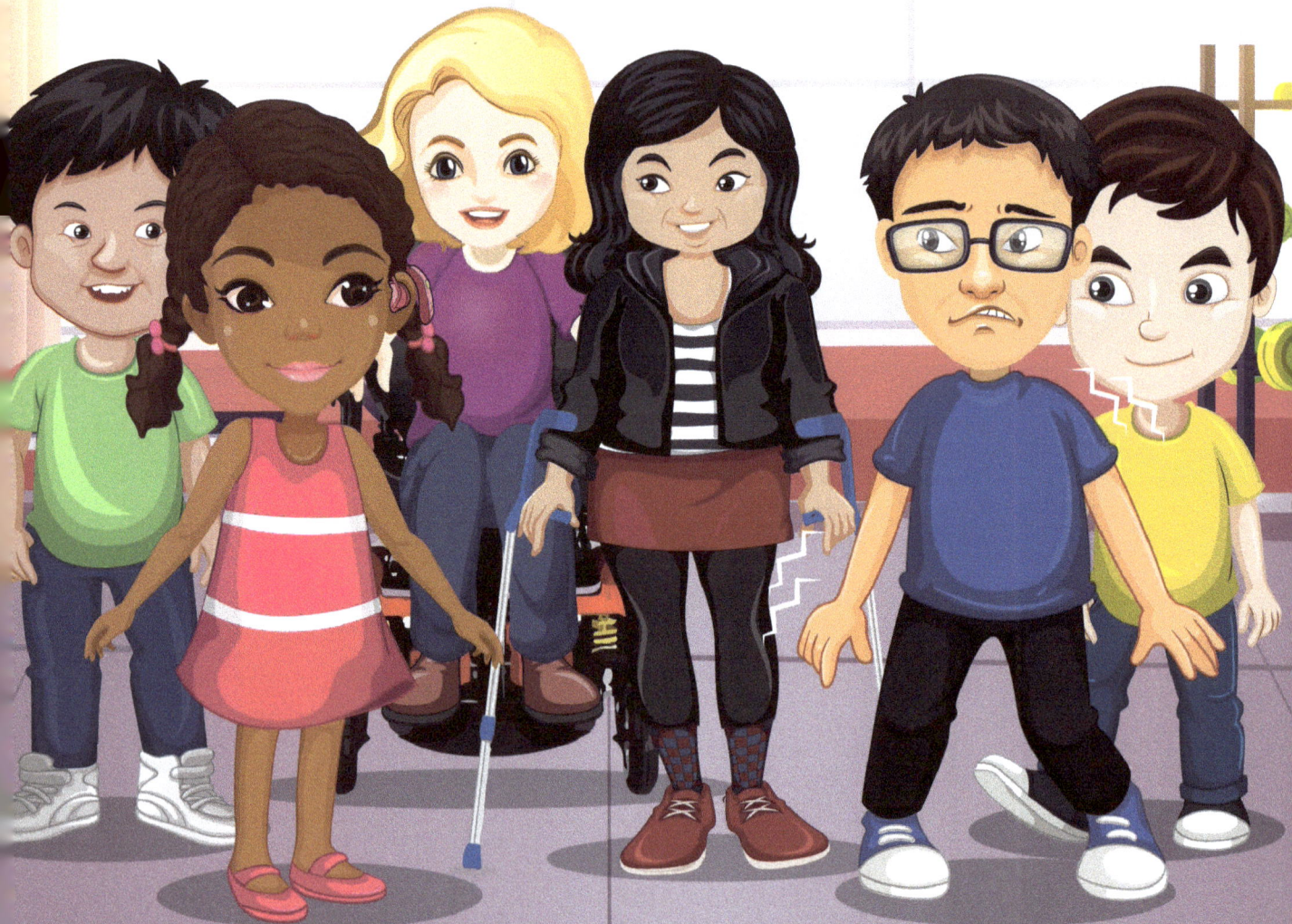

Mrs. Rosie grabbed Emmanuel by the hand and said "everyone, this is Emmanuel " He is not much for words or or making small talk. Some people may say that's his weakness.

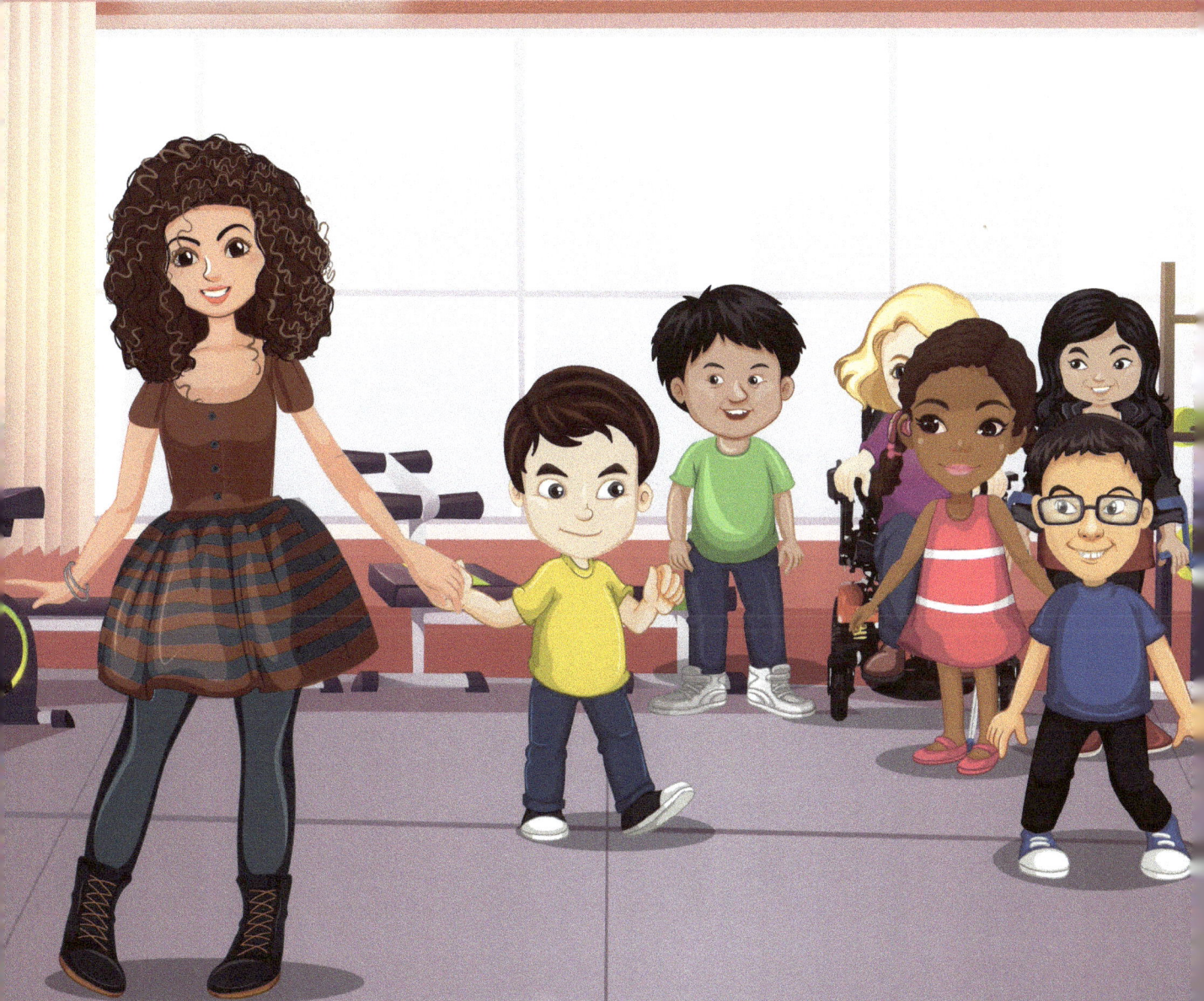

On the flip side, he has Autism and that means even if you don't always hear him he is always listening, watching everything around him and understands most things and that's his superpower.

Very quietly strolled in Maci in her motor chair.

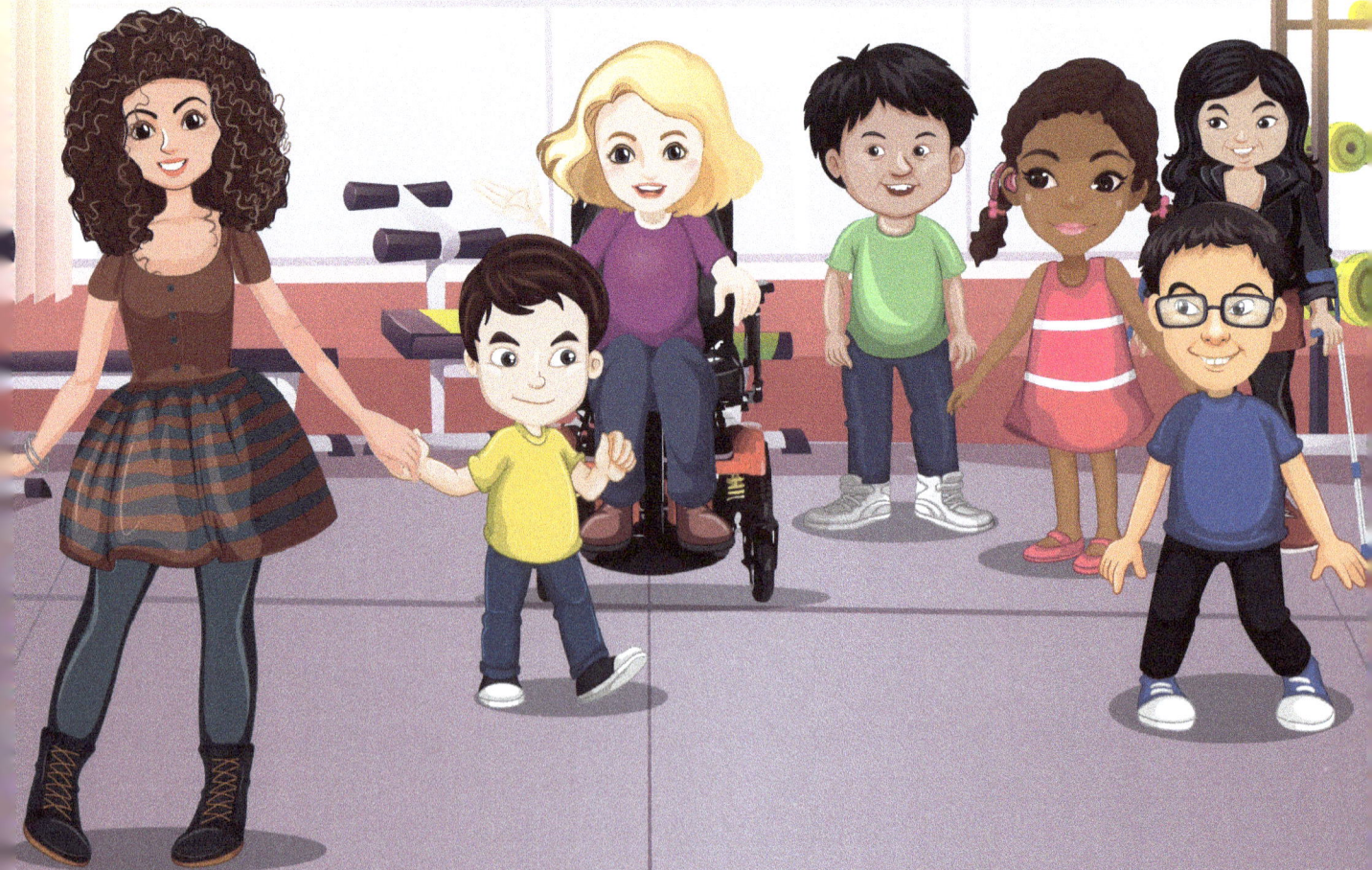

She stood up off her motor chair and walked across the area. On her way back to the motor chair she said "I have Muscular Dystrophy and it hurts to do normal things like walking."

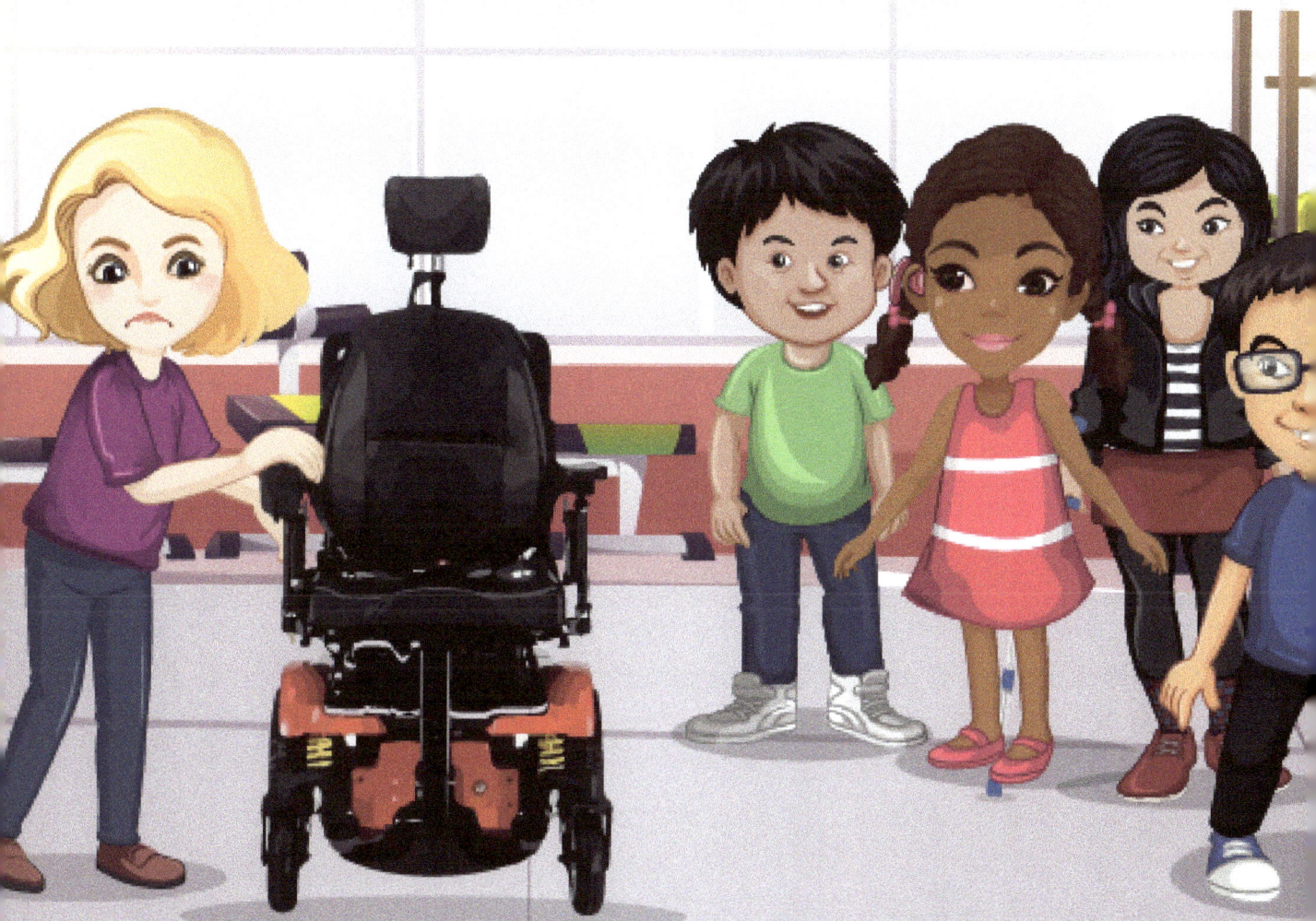

When I can walk it's my superpower and my weakness is when I get sad about what I was born with because their is no cure for my condition..

Aj knew he had to say his part now, not only was it his turn but it was just the right time.

Aj wanted Maci to know that he will be her friend and and she never has to feel sad again.  Aj said his super power is that no matter what Doctors told him he wouldn't do a lot of things like most of you, or live a long life and guess what?

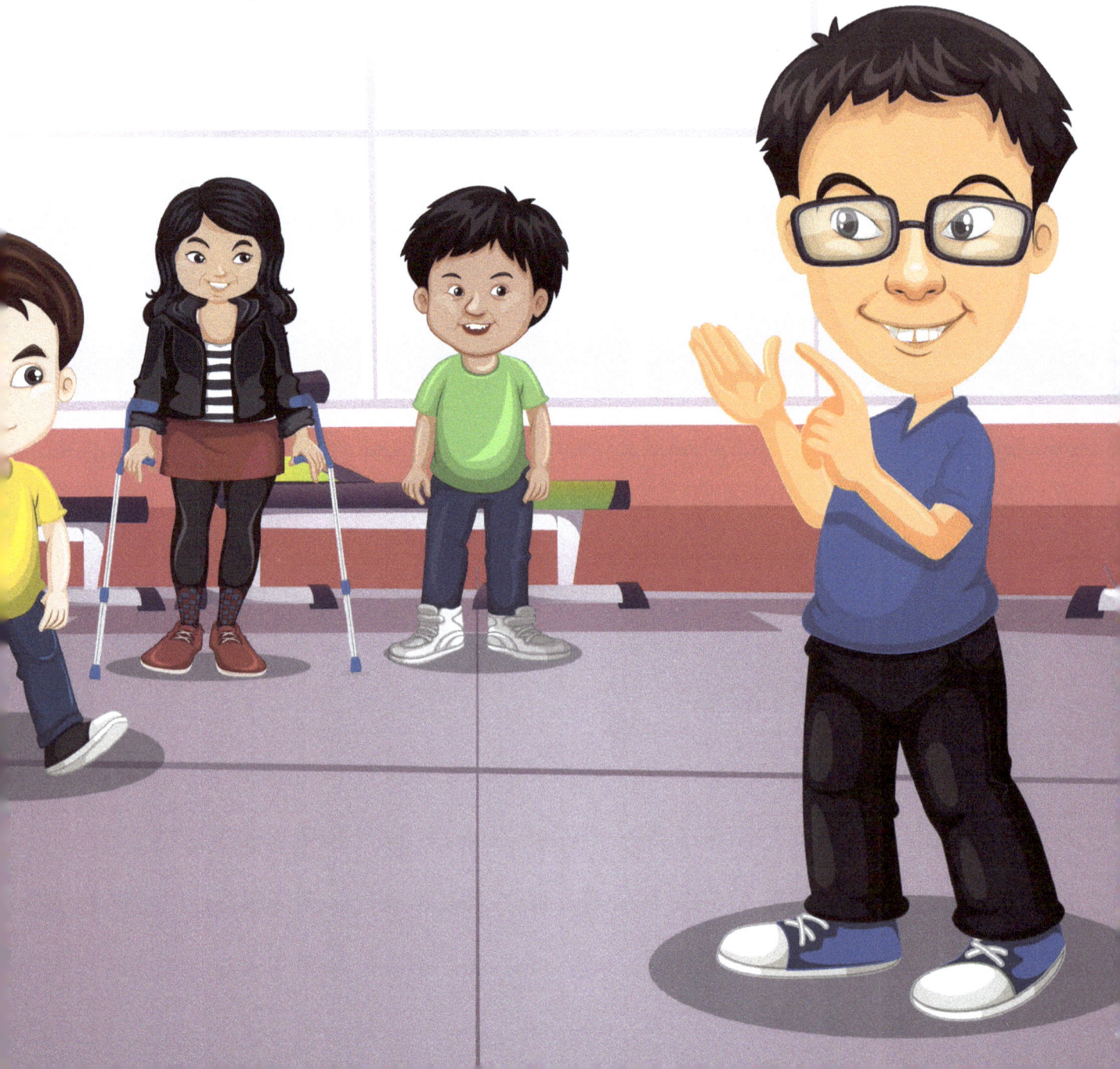

Aj was so happy to say his part he started to flap his hands and said "I don't, I live a better than normal with a smile I push myself every day." My weakness is not having a name to my disability. It's so rare I'm like a really cool medical unicorn.

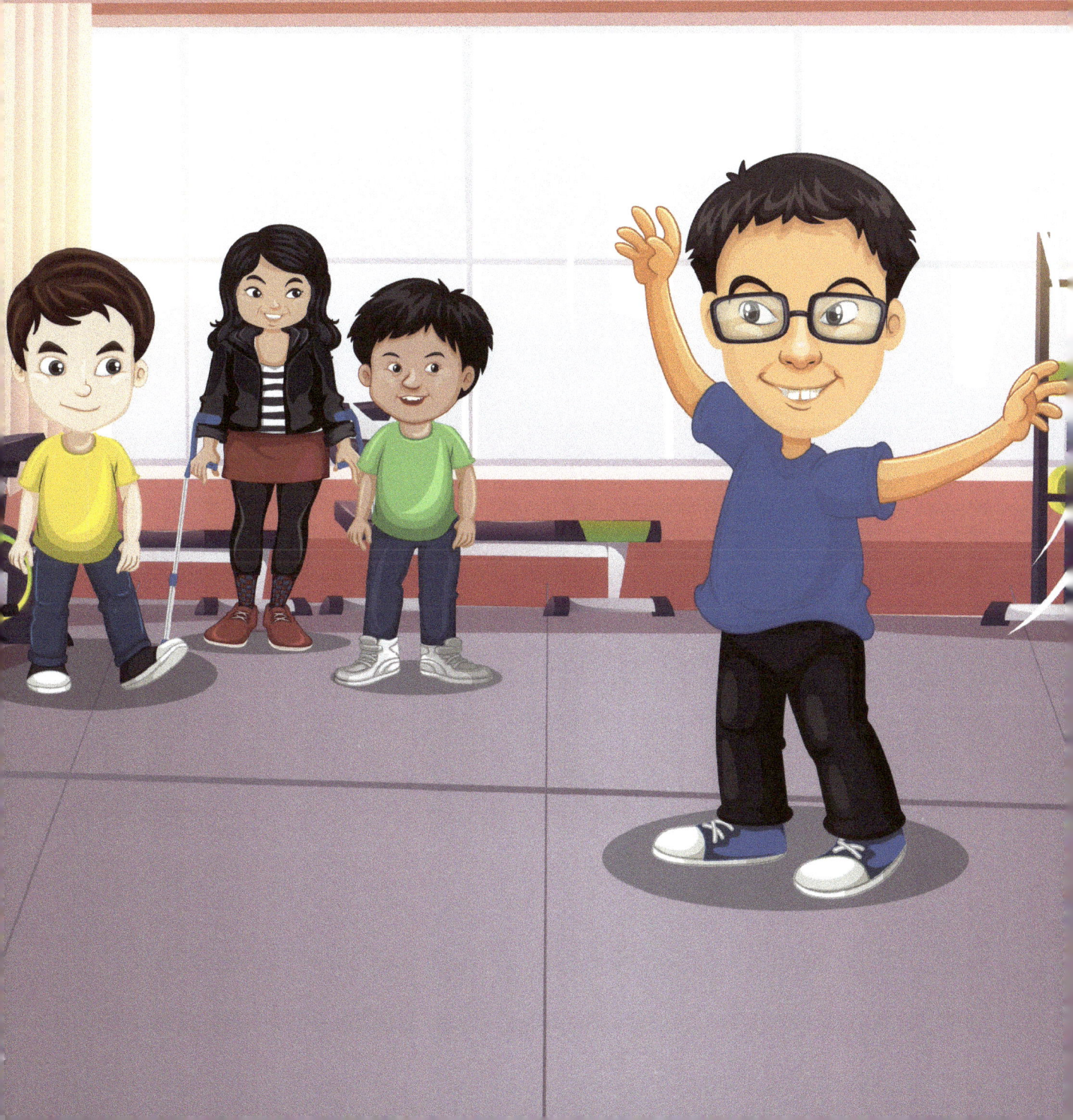

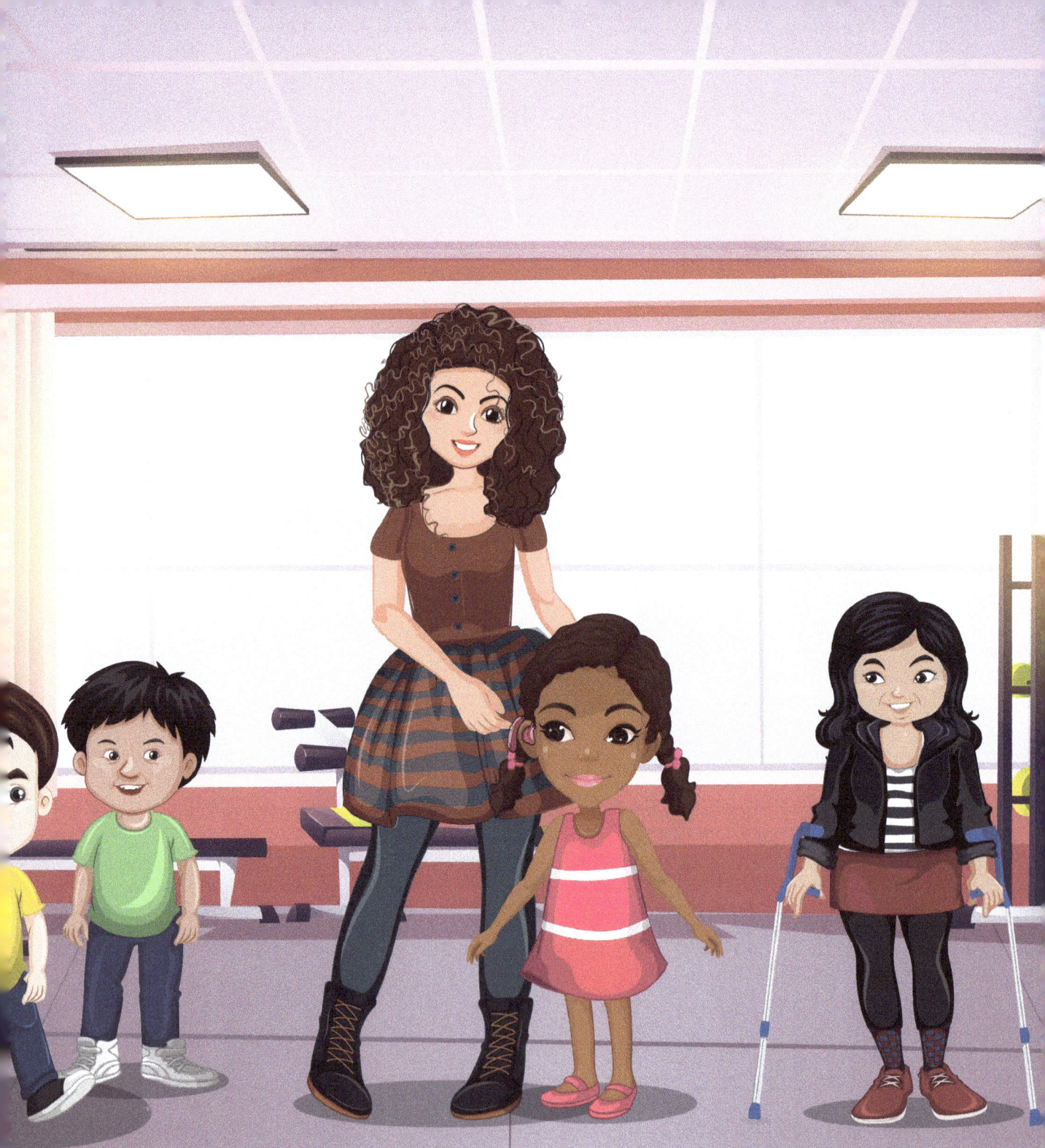

Mrs. Rosie was so proud of her group she even had tears in her eyes. Imani came towards Mrs. Rosie and hugged her.

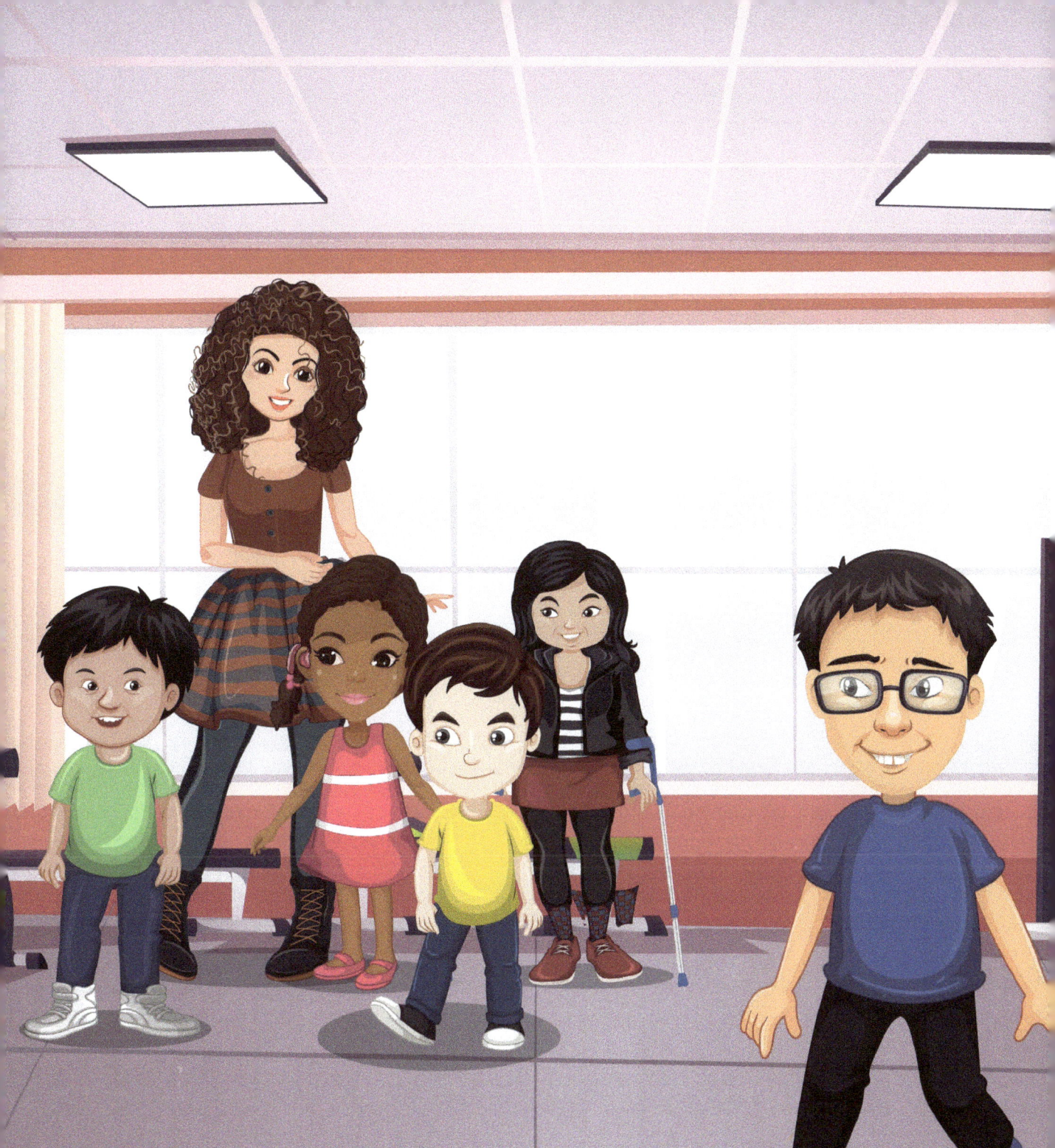

Aj looked around and felt good like this was
going to be a great week.
Aj felt like he already made friends.

Jesse stood in front of the group and said "so does this mean we all have a weakness and a disability?"

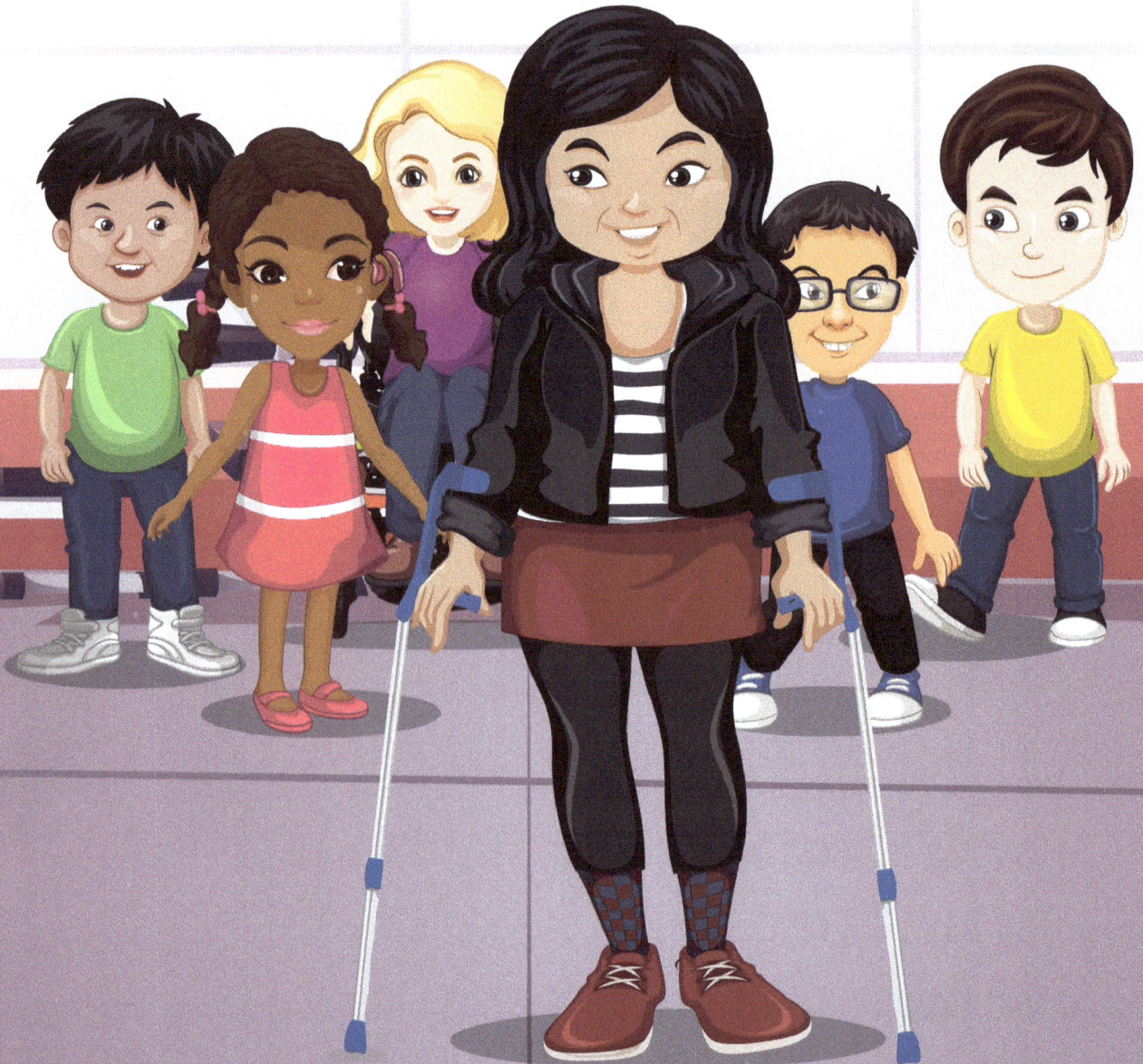

Mrs. Rosie said I like to say that this camp is full of superpowers and kids with abilities. So now that we know what they are let's enjoy the week.

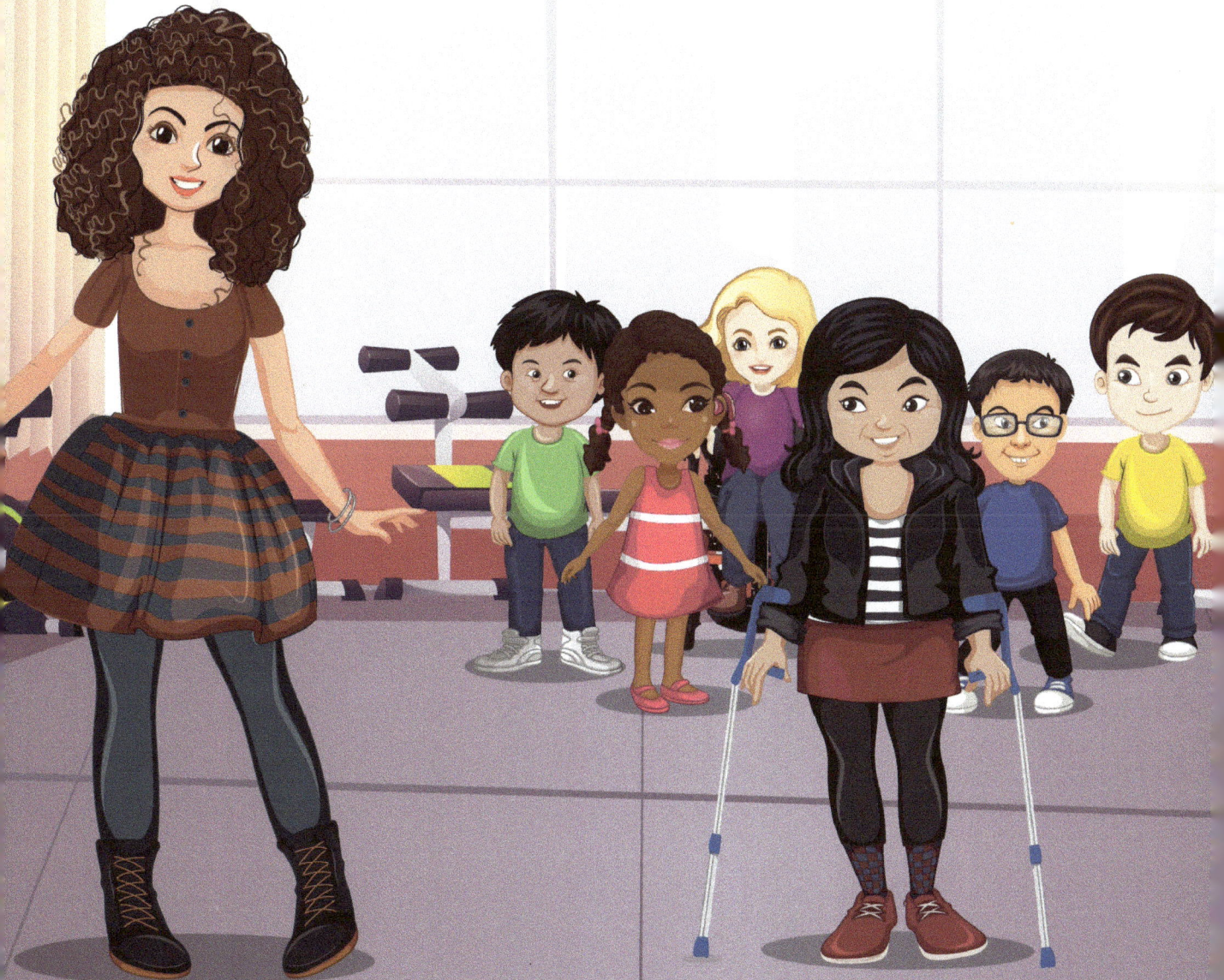

The next few days the kids played, did arts and crafts. They made yummy gooey smores while telling stories by the camp fires.

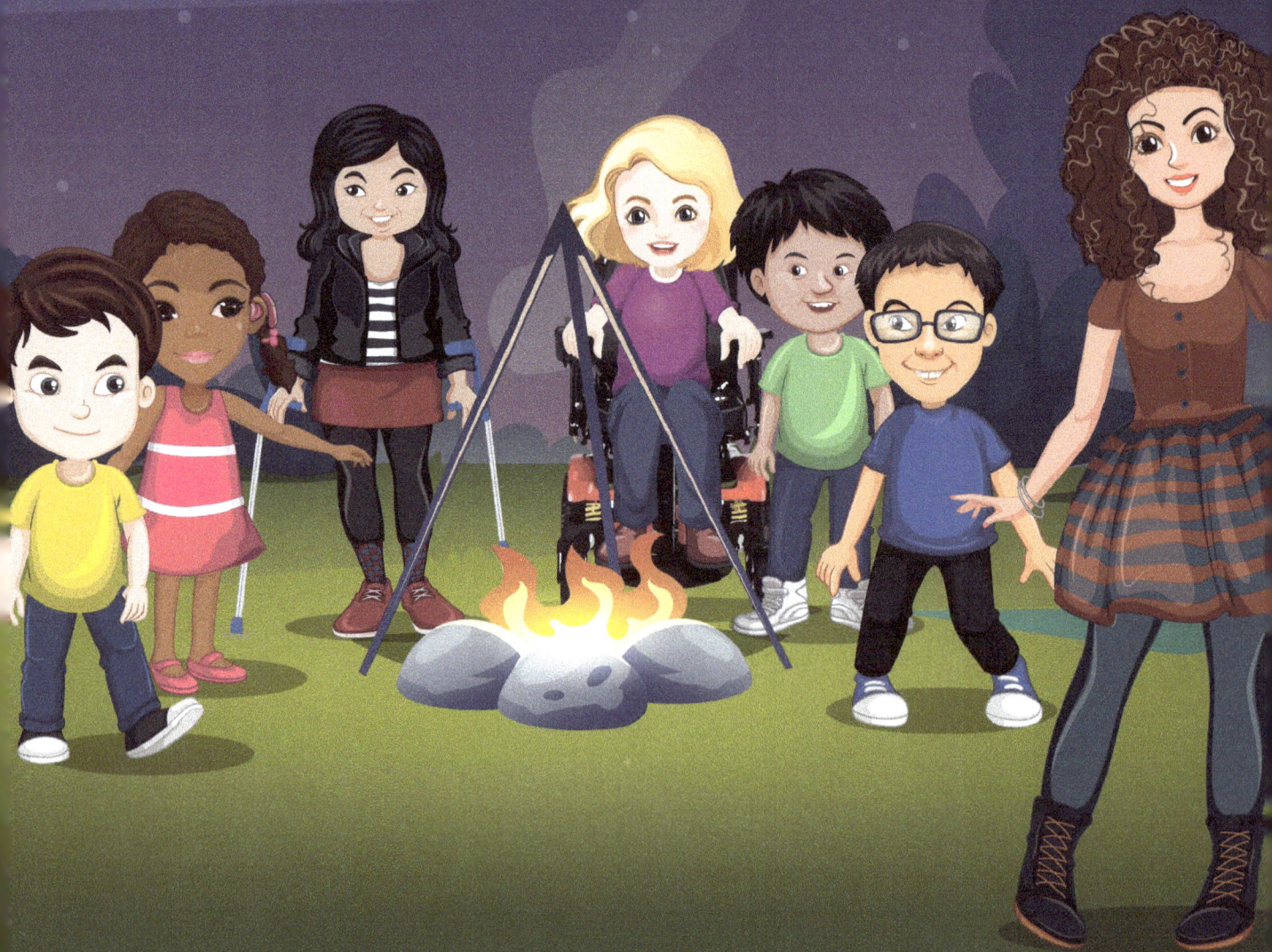

On the final day the camp held their field day for all the kids. Mrs. Rosie had made special t-shirts with her group during craft time. The group came up with the name Superstar Heroes after Aj told everyone he is Superstar Aj.

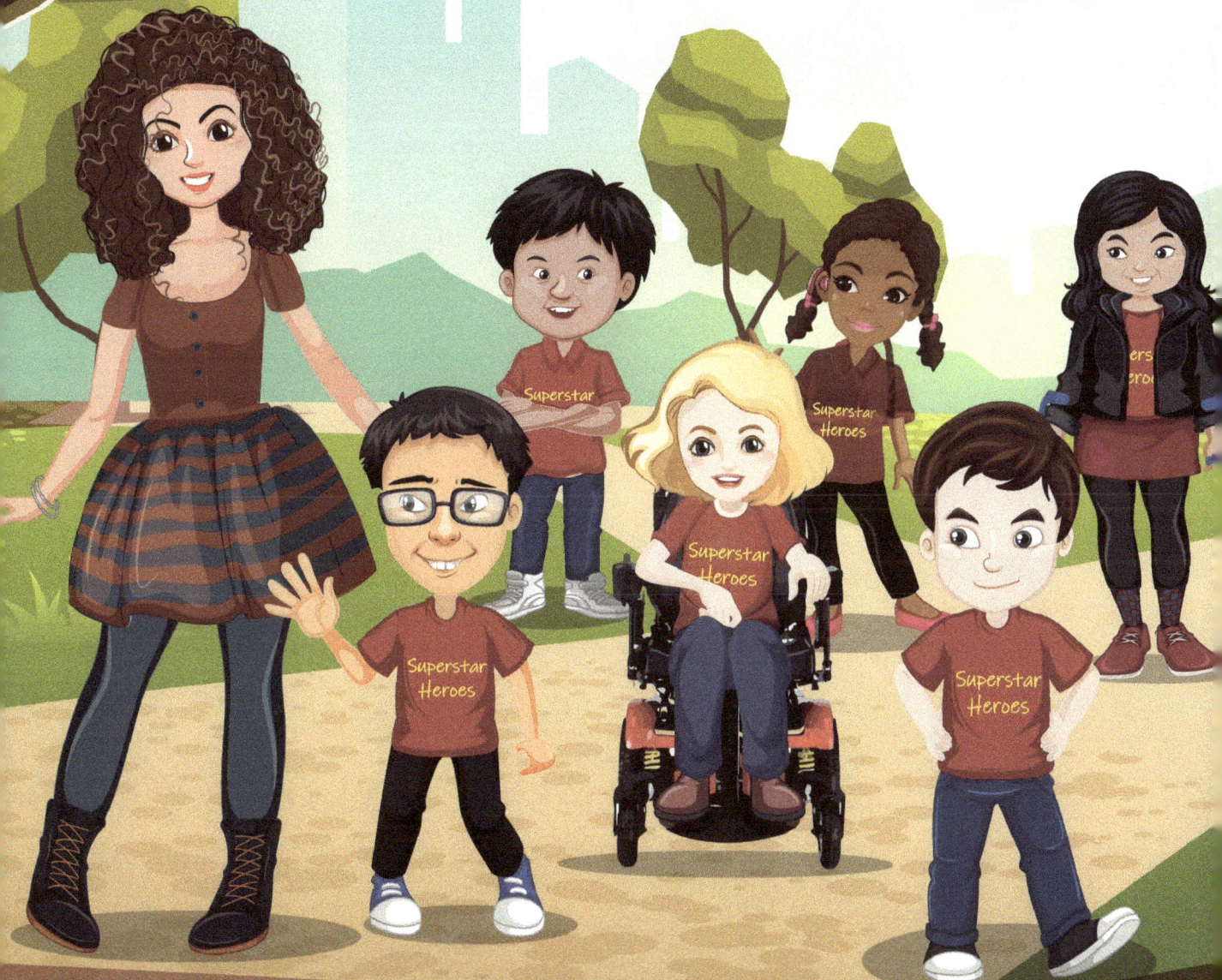

The games at field day had musical chairs which Danny won since he was fast and loved music.

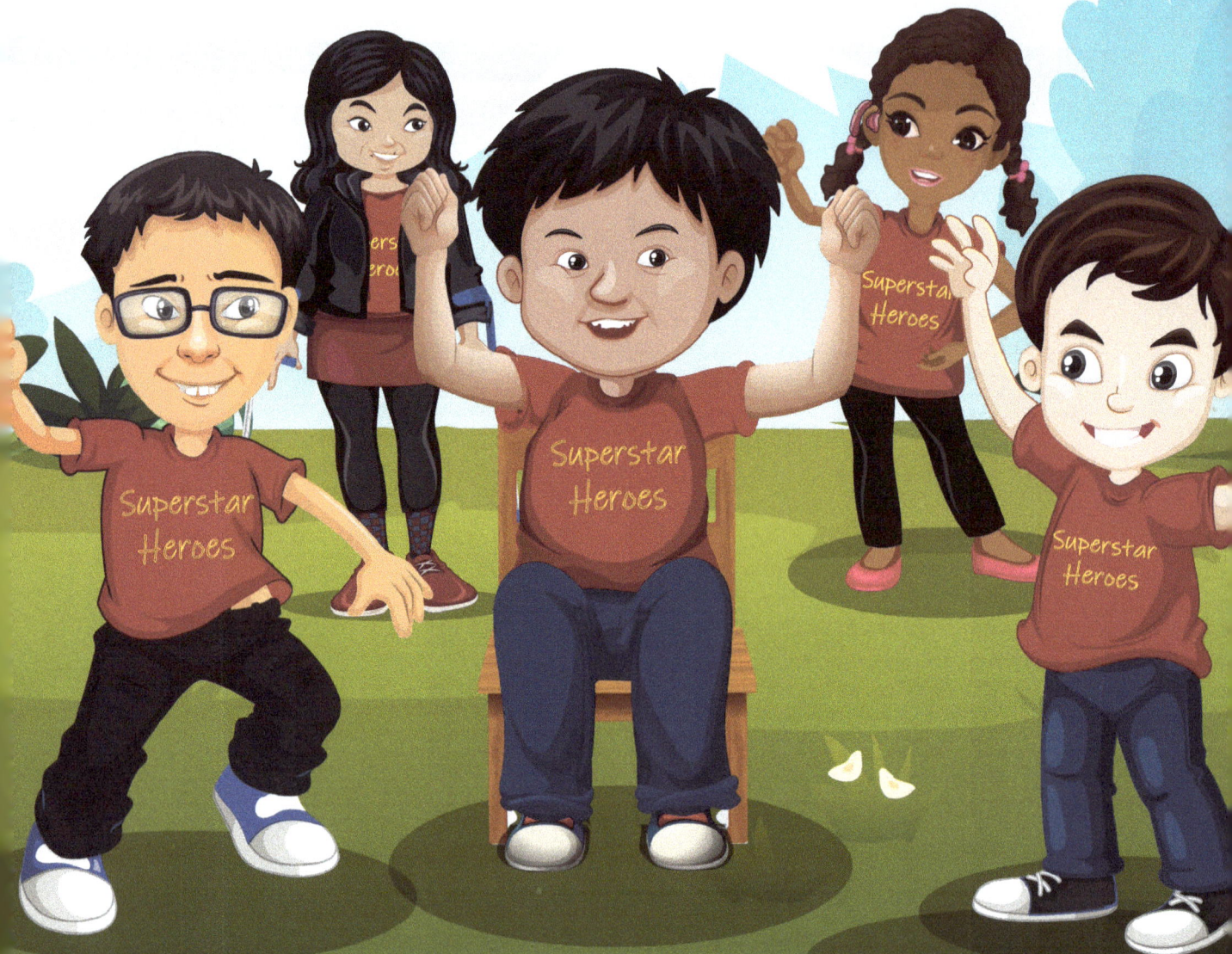

A blind course where Jessie used her voice to guide Imani who listened to the finish line first.

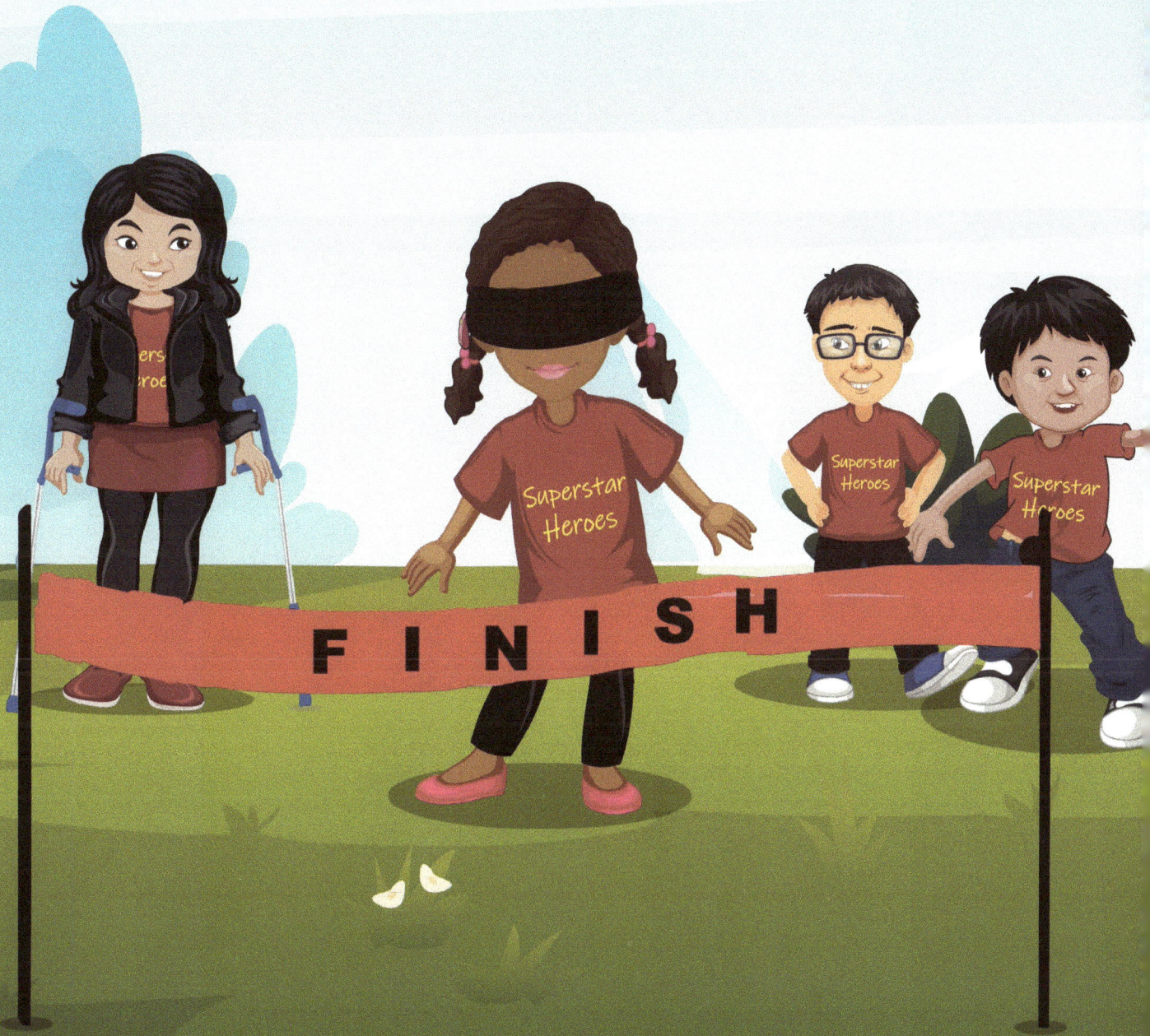

Maci's motor chair was the fastest when it came to moving all the toys from one box to another and the Superstars had won that game too.

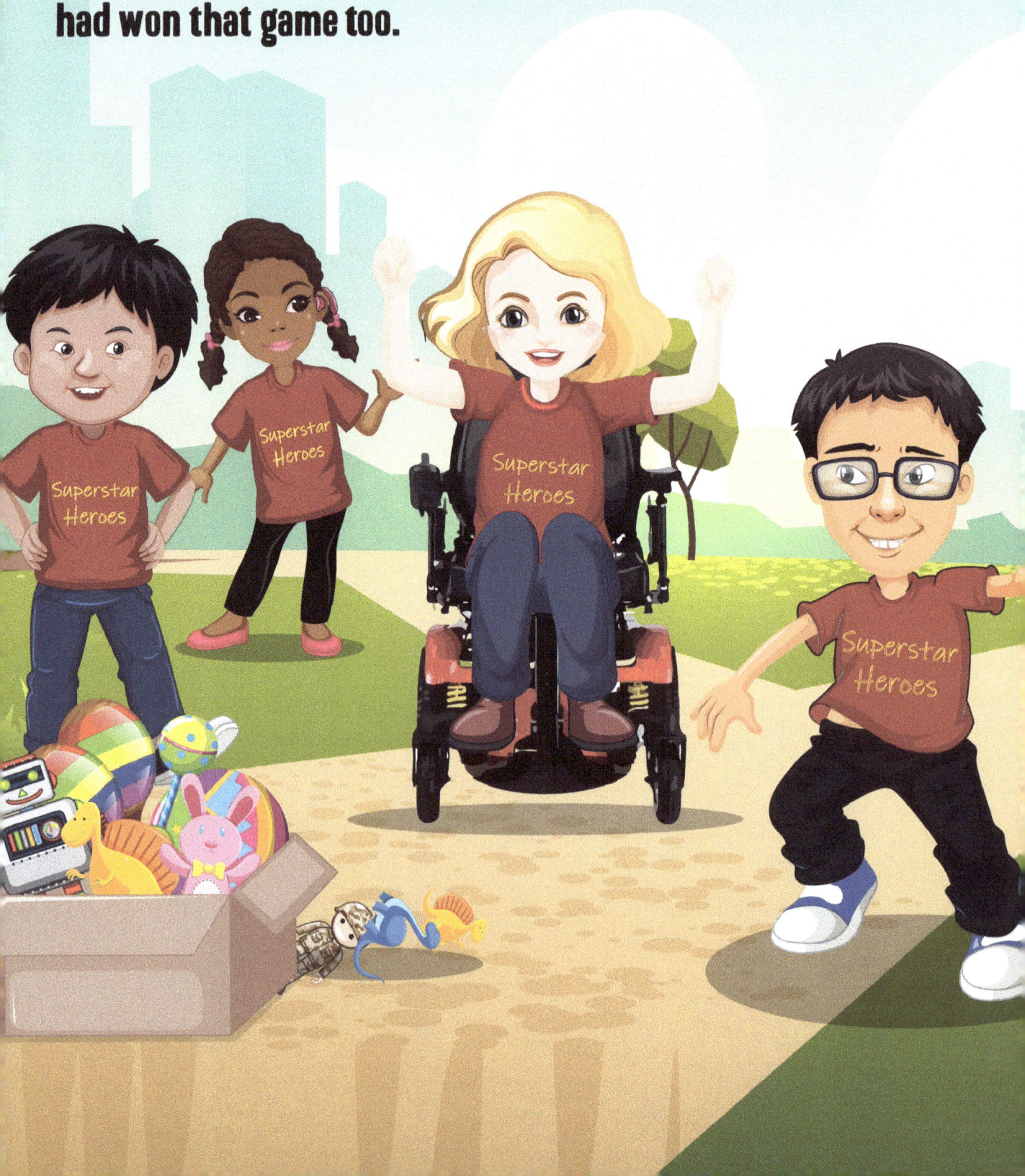

A puzzle had to be solved and Emmanuel was perfect for the job. He loves puzzles and he was so good at it. He won that game and shouted "I won I'm so happy" everyone was filled with joy hearing him speak.

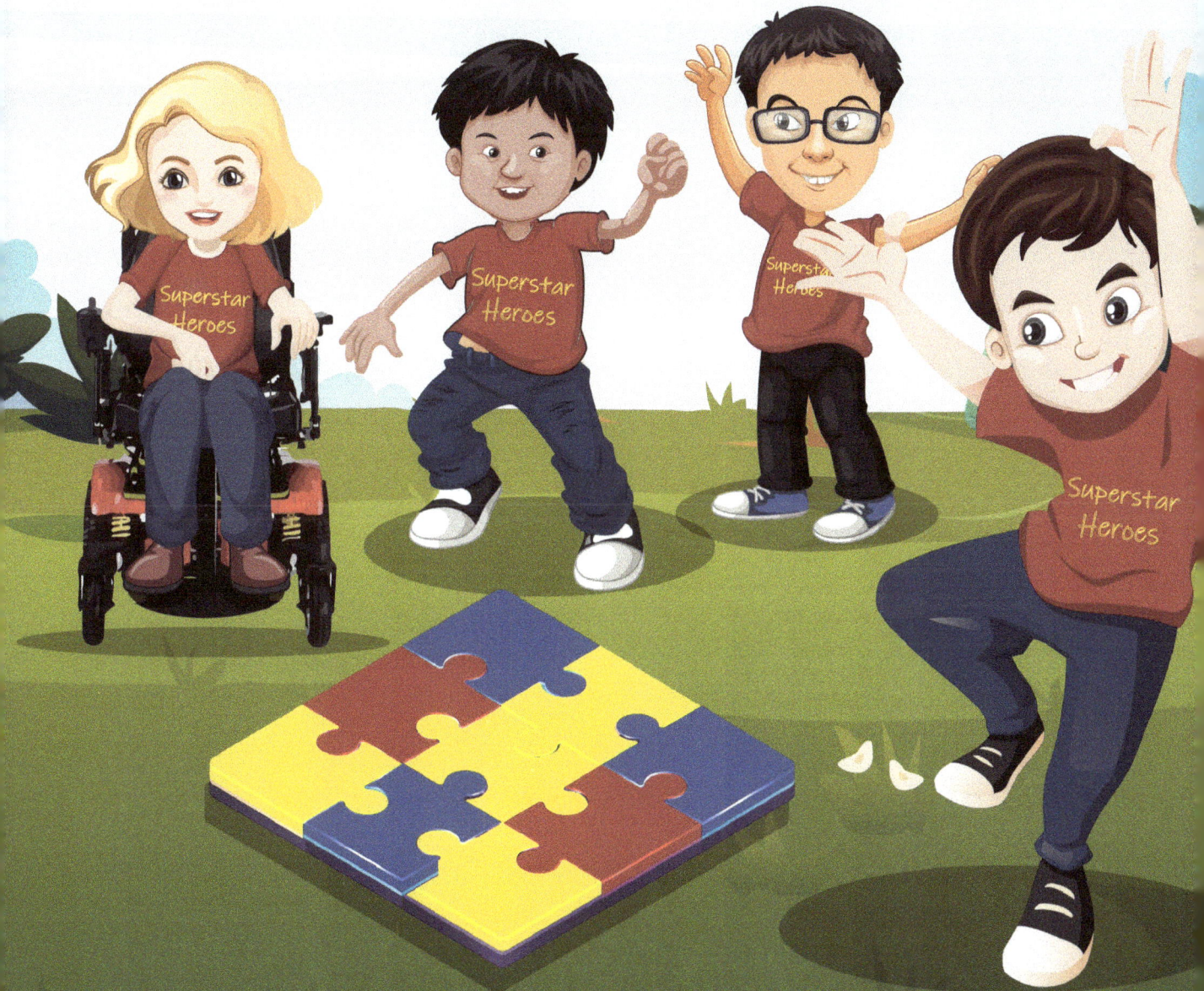

All the kids were smiling from ear to ear happy to be at this camp and a part of this team. The last game was an obstacle course.

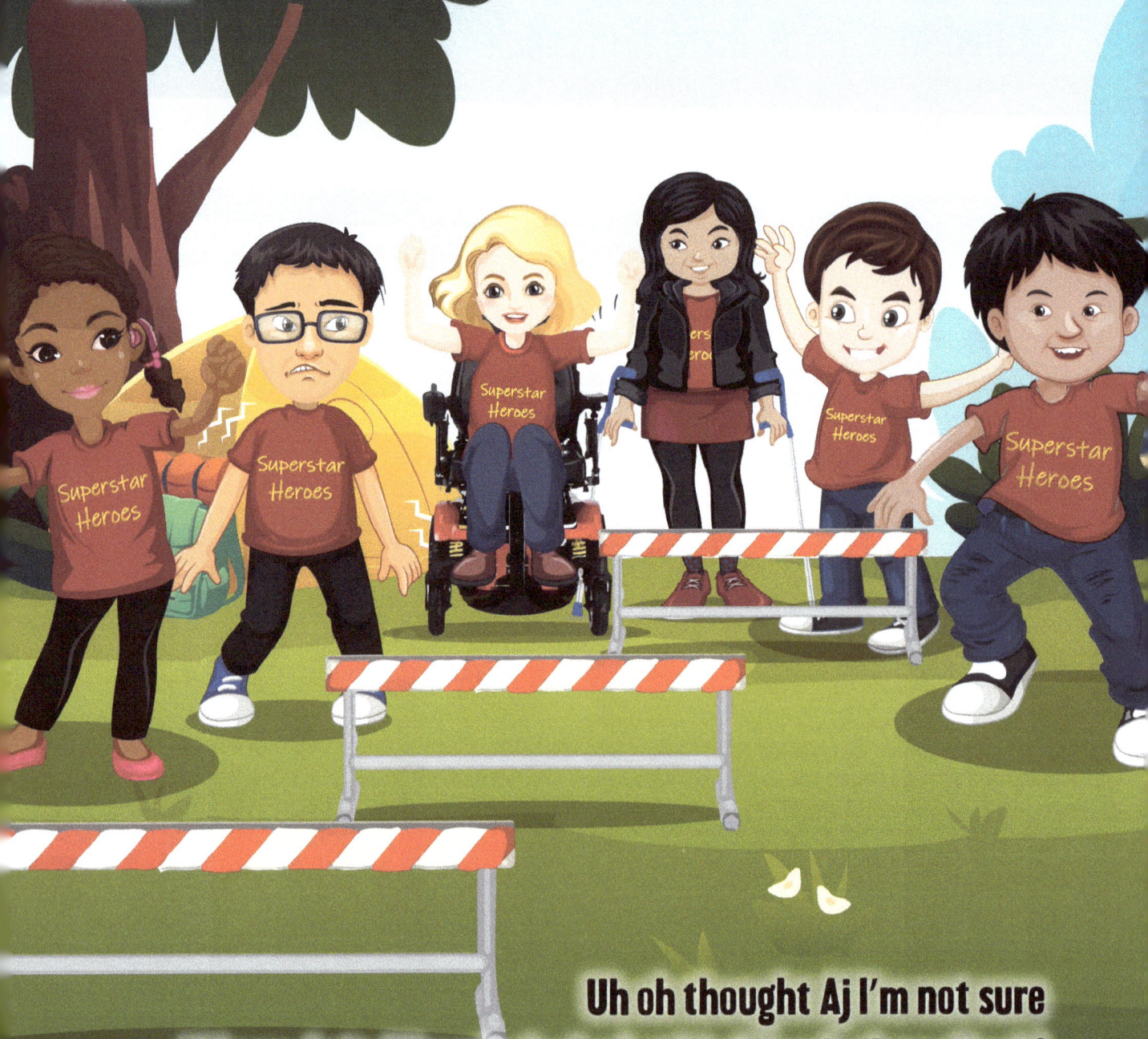

Uh oh thought Aj I'm not sure if I can do it. When he looked at his friends they all said Aj you got this just like the first day of camp.

You're Superstar Aj. Aj ran the course fast which was so hard he crawled under the ropes climbed the small hill and made it to the end. He was out of breath with his hands on his knees he took some deep breaths and then he needed to use his asthma pump to get some air. He felt so tired but he won he did it.

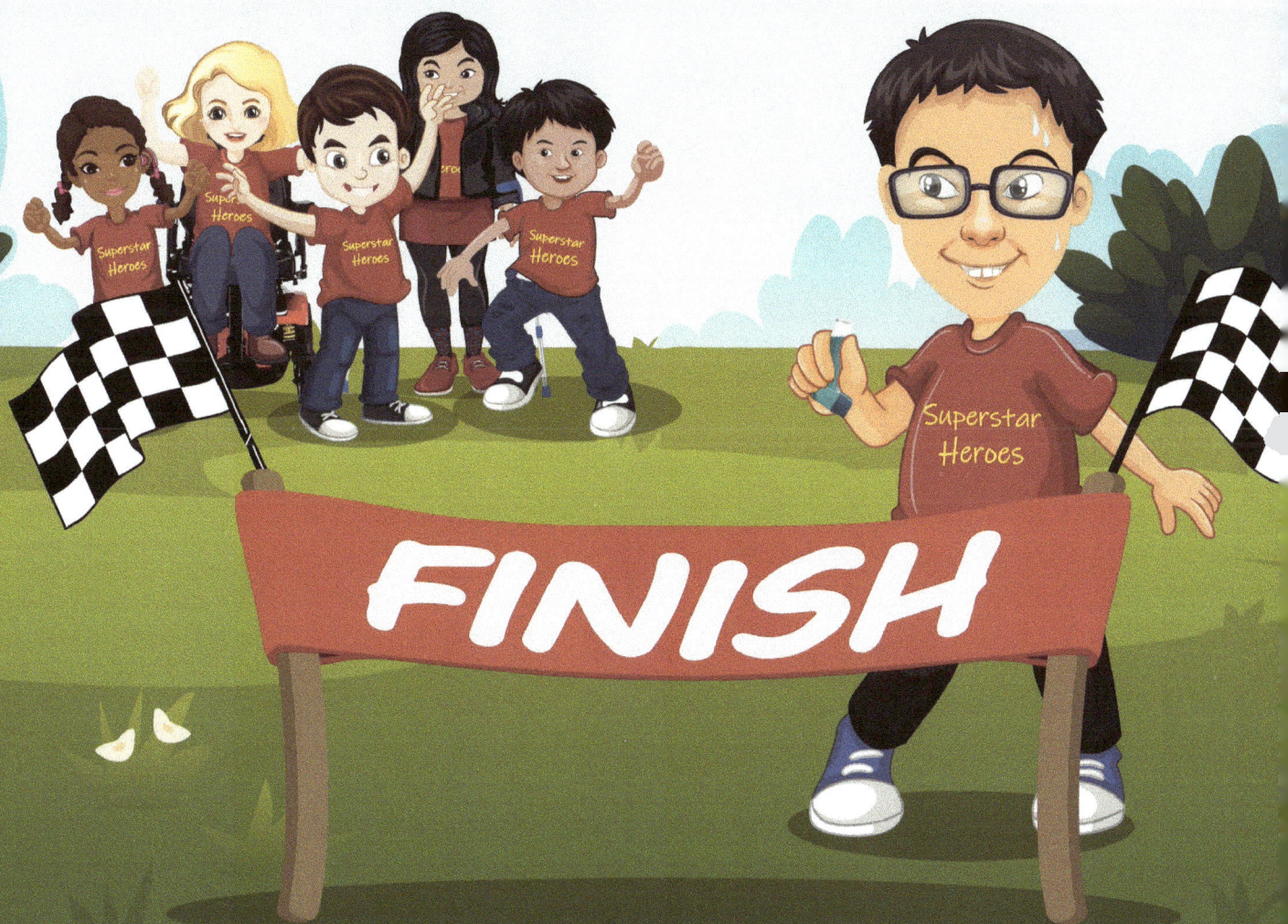

FINISH

Superstars all did it. The camp gave everyone a trophy for trying their very best.

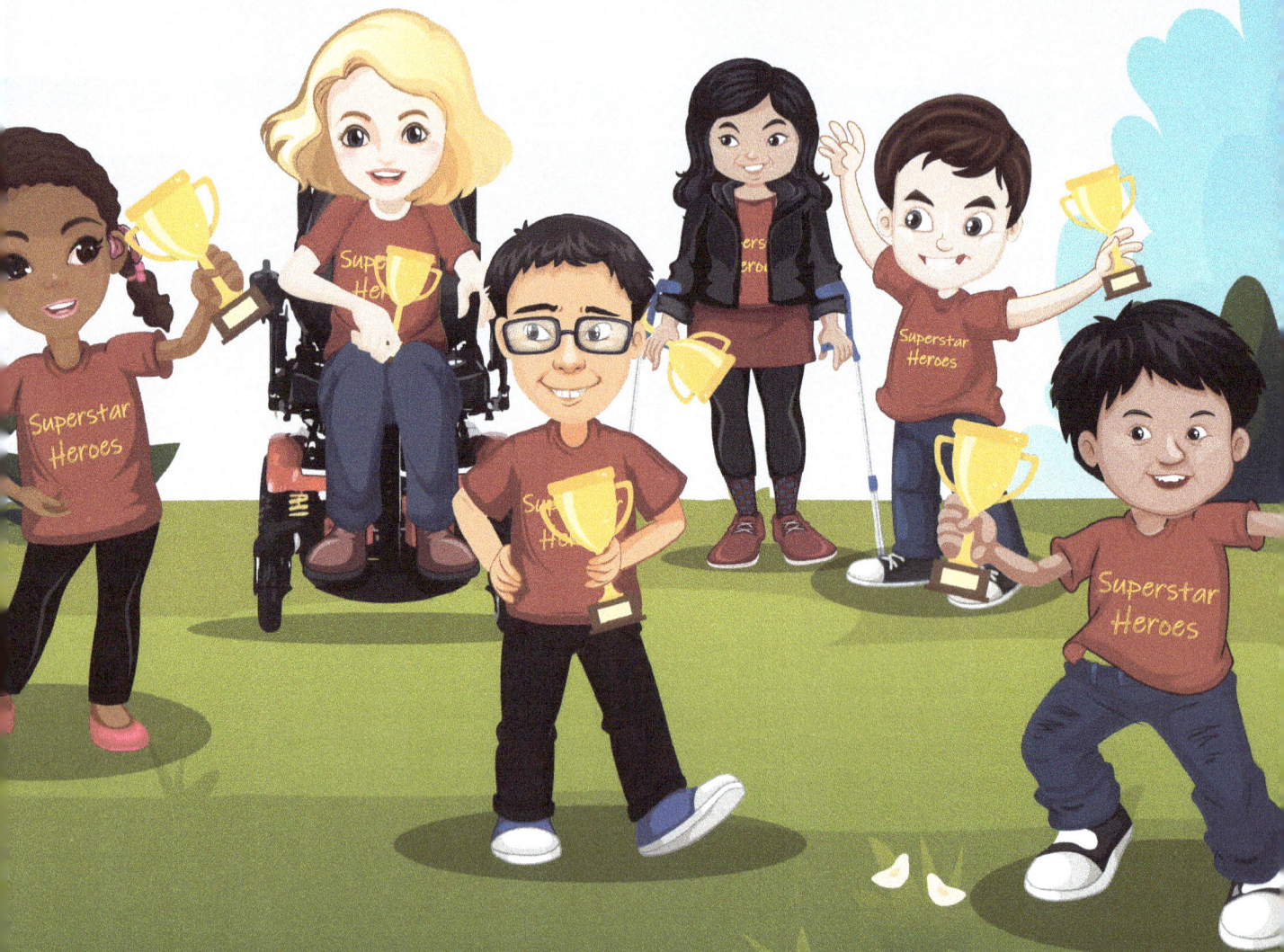

They had a party with music cake and lots of pictures. Mrs. Rosie loves to take pictures and so she did all week for family and friends.

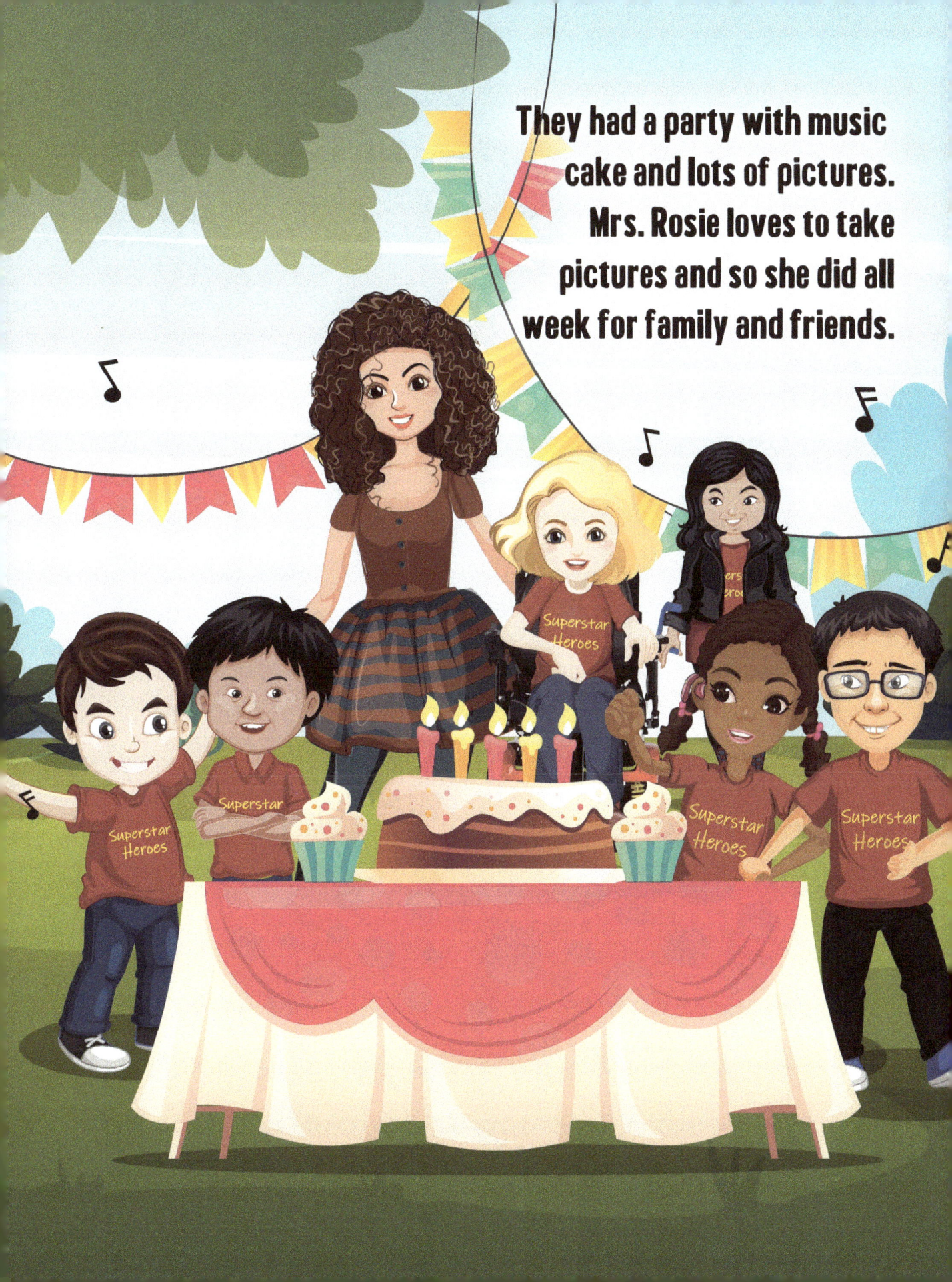

Time has come to say goodbye, said Mrs. Rosie. Aj said it's never goodbye it's see you later. We are all friends now and can't wait for the next adventure.

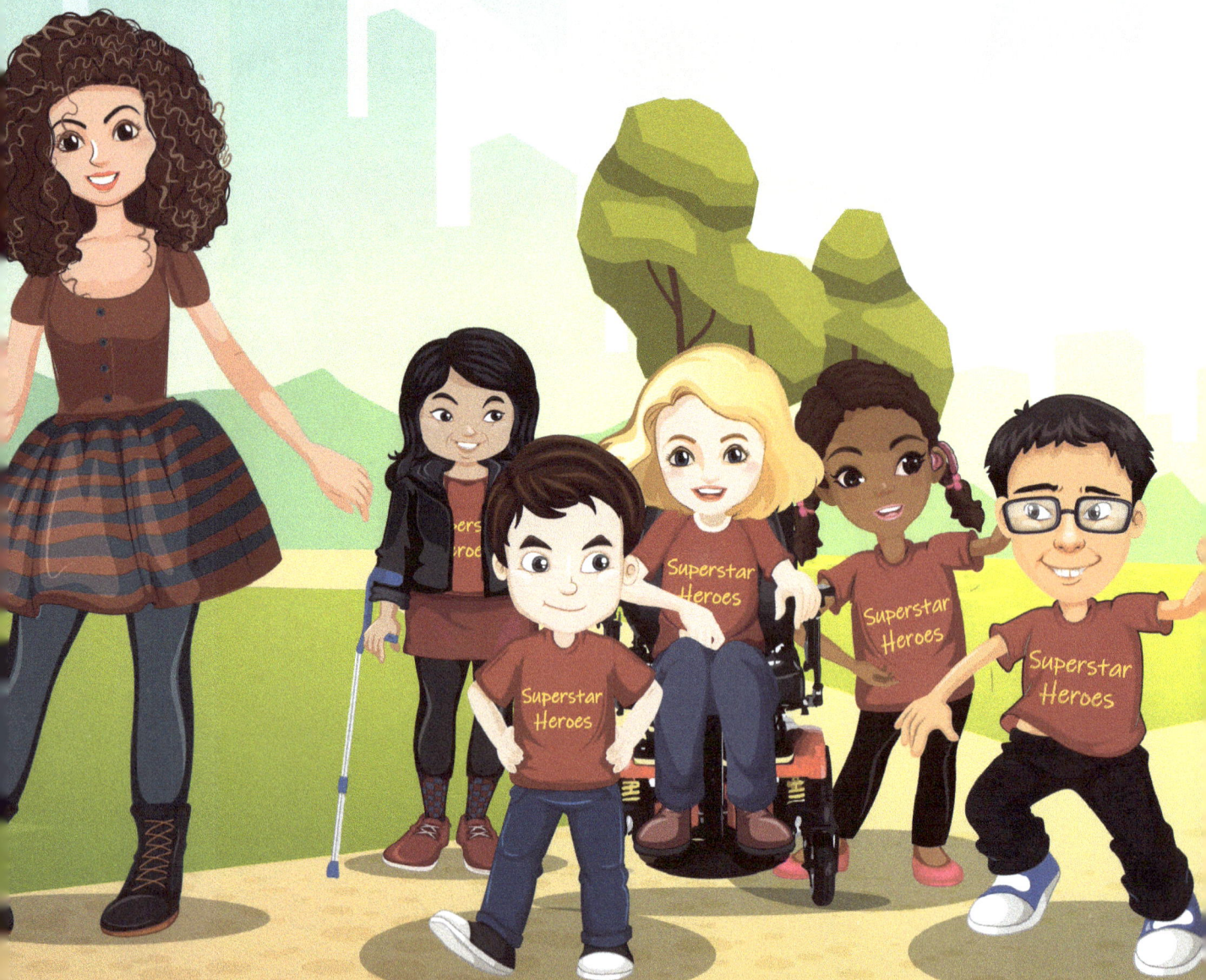

Everyone laughed because Aj always had something to say from the first day to the last day.

When AJ reached home his big brother Ethan was so happy to see him. Ethan waited outside to hug his brother.
Aj said I missed you but I made cool new friends let me tell you all about the Superstar Heroes.

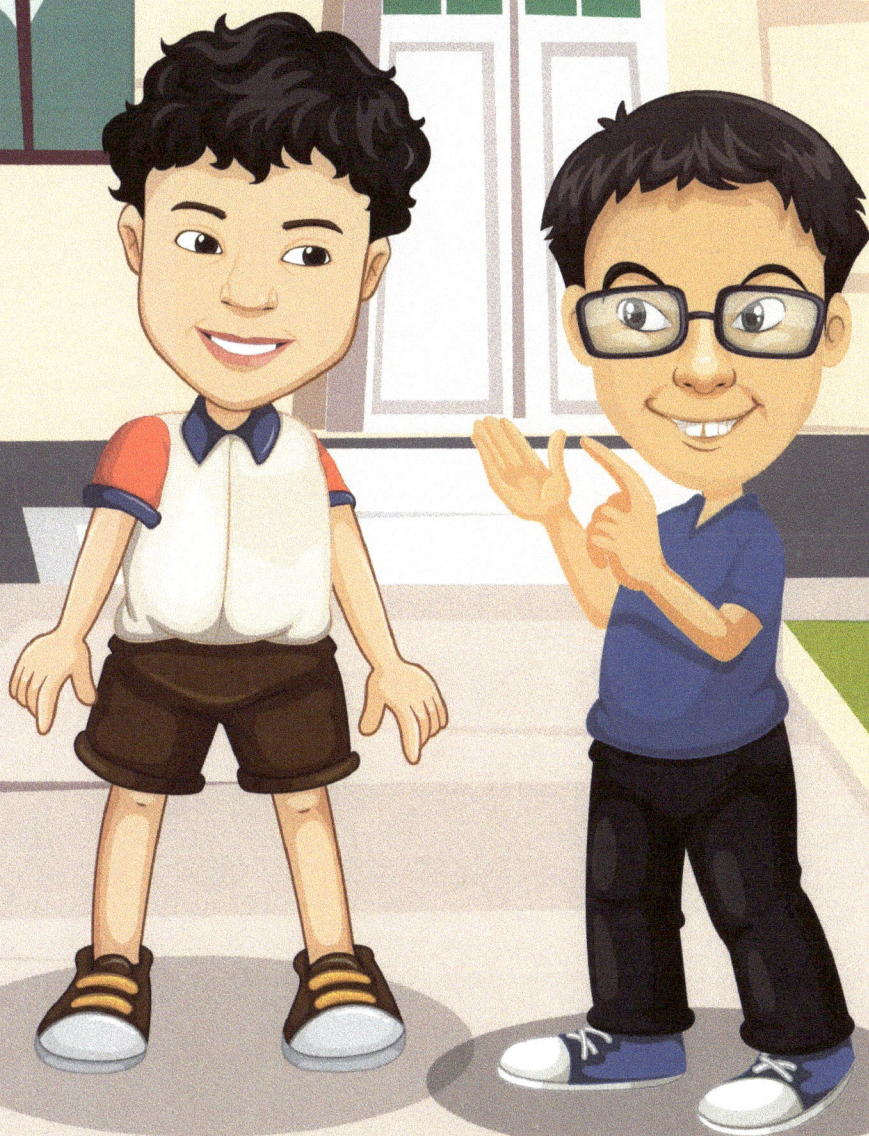

# Autism

Where a child may think and understand differently than a typical child. Learning may also be different for a autistic child. Talking and interacting may not come easy to a child with Autism. Autistic children senses are used more and that will make a child more sensitive to things like sounds and textures to touch.

1 out of every 54 kids are diagnosed with Autsim Spectrum Disorder.

https://nationalautismassociation.org/resources/autism-fact-sheet/

# Cerebral Palsy

When your brain has a hard time communicating with your muscles, So talking, walking and even eating are hard. 10,000 kids are born yearly with CP.

https://www.cerebralpalsyguidance.com/cerebral-palsy/research/facts-and-statistics/

# Deafness/Hearing Loss

To hear very little or nothing at all.
From birth or can get worse over time.
2-3 children out every 1,000 births are
born with hearing loss.

https://www.nidcd.nih.gov/health/statistics/quick-statistics-hearing

# Down Syndrome

Children born with Down Syndrome physically have similar eye shape where the eye slants up. Down syndrome children may be born with heart problems or have problems as they grow. Children with this syndrome have a hard time learning and need more help with self care.

About 1 in every 700 babies are born with down syndrome.

# Muscular Dystrophy

Muscular dystrophy is a group of muscle diseases where the muscles in the body become weak and get weaker as the child grows. The muscle breaks down and it is hard to walk until they can no longer walk.

Usually by the age of 12, the child needs a wheelchair because the leg muscles are too weak to work.

www.Childrenswi.org/medical-care/neuroscience/conditions/muscular-dystrophy

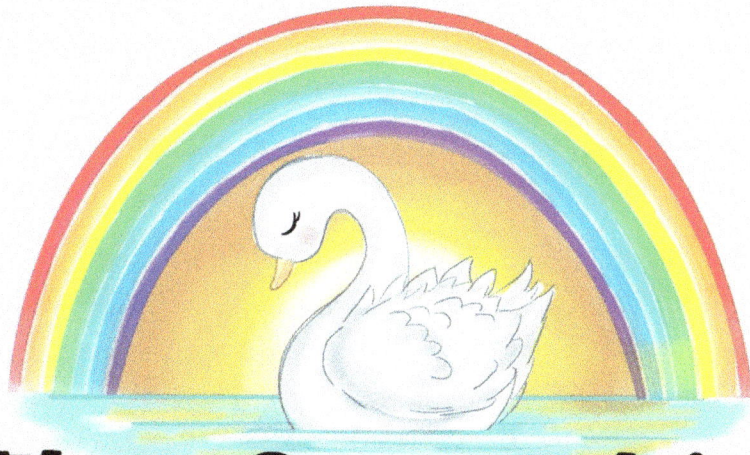

# Syndrome Without A Name (S.W.A.N)

**A person born with atypical features, conditions but there has been no test to confirm a specific syndrome because the lack of information or cases.**

www.ingramcontent.com/pod-product-compliance
Lightning Source LLC
Chambersburg PA
CBHW041055050426
42335CB00057B/3336